Program Evaluation

This timely, unique, and insightful book provides students and practitioners with the tools and skills needed to evaluate social and policy programs across a range of disciplines—from public health to social work to education—enabling the allocation of scarce human and financial resources to advance the health and well-being of individuals and populations.

The chapters are organized according to the main tasks involved in conducting an evaluation to produce unbiased evidence of program effectiveness, quality, and value. The chapters include methods for selecting and justifying evaluation questions or hypotheses, designing evaluations, sampling participants, selecting information sources, and ensuring reliable and valid measurement. The final section of the book is focused on managing and analyzing data and transparently reporting the results in written and oral form. The book features international case studies throughout, covers quantitative, qualitative, and mixed-method approaches, and is also informed by new online methods developed during the COVID-19 pandemic. Among the book's unique features is a focus on international standards for conducting ethical evaluations and avoiding research misconduct.

Also featuring checklists, example forms, and summaries of the key ideas and topics, this very practical book is essential reading for students in the social, behavioral, and health sciences, and will be a key resource for professionals in the field.

Arlene Fink, Ph.D., is Professor of Medicine and Public Health at the University of California, Los Angeles, USA. She is an expert in program evaluation, survey research, and research methodology found at the intersection of public health and medicine. She has conducted and advised on more than 40 program evaluations in numerous fields from education to medicine and has lectured nationally and internationally. Dr. Fink is the author of more than 130 peer-reviewed articles and ten textbooks.

T0372801

Program Evaluation

A Primer for Effectiveness, Quality, and Value

Arlene Fink

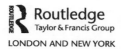

Routledge
Taylor & Francis Group

LONDON AND NEW YORK

Designed cover image: © Getty Images

First published 2024
by Routledge
4 Park Square, Milton Park, Abingdon, Oxon OX14 4RN

and by Routledge
605 Third Avenue, New York, NY 10158

Routledge is an imprint of the Taylor & Francis Group, an informa business

© 2024 Arlene Fink

British Library Cataloguing-in-Publication Data
A catalogue record for this book is available from the British Library

ISBN: 978-1-032-63506-4 (hbk)
ISBN: 978-1-032-36787-3 (pbk)
ISBN: 978-1-032-63507-1 (ebk)

DOI: 10.4324/9781032635071

Typeset in Times New Roman
by KnowledgeWorks Global Ltd.

This book is dedicated to the ones I love: John C. Beck, Gretel, Ingrid, Anja, Astrid, Daniella, and Ingvard.

CONTENTS

Chapter 4. Sampling in Program Evaluations

Chapter 8. Analyzing Evaluation Data

Chapter 9. Evaluation Reports

LIST OF FIGURES

LIST OF TABLES

LIST OF EXAMPLES

CHAPTER 1 | INTRODUCING PROGRAM EVALUATION

An evaluation is a systematic assessment of a program's effectiveness, quality, and value. High-quality evaluations are scientific studies that result in unbiased evidence of the program's achievements, impact, and costs. Stakeholders use evaluation information to better understand their program and to make informed decisions about program improvement, continuation, and funding.

An effective program achieves positive outcomes and provides measurable benefits to its targeted population. In an effective program, the benefits are greater than their human and financial costs. A high-quality program meets its stakeholders' needs and is based on sound theory and the best available research evidence. A program's value is measured by its costs and worth to its stakeholders, the community, and society. Each program evaluation must decide whether it will investigate effectiveness, quality, or value—or all three, a decision sometimes made jointly with stakeholders.

This chapter explains the methods that evaluators use to obtain unbiased evidence of a program's effectiveness, quality, and value. The chapter gives examples of program evaluations and describes their purposes, methods, and stakeholders and provides guidance for preventing bias. The chapter also discusses formative and summative evaluations, qualitative and mixed-methods research, and stakeholder engagement in participatory and collaborative evaluations. The chapter introduces comparative and cost-effectiveness evaluations and describes their methods and importance. Sometimes a scientific study is unlikely. The chapter discusses how to provide a systematic program assessment and describes its limitations. The chapter also provides examples of program evaluation frameworks that can be used to structure the evaluation process.

Many program evaluations, particularly randomized and non-randomized studies, include human subjects. Increasingly, program evaluators are asked to state in their report whether their evaluations measure up to ethical principles for doing human subjects' research. Funding agencies and many journals in all fields will only accept reports that provide evidence that the evaluation was reviewed and approved by an ethics board. The chapter discusses how to conduct and report on evaluations that follow internationally accepted ethics principles by respecting the uniqueness and independence of individuals, securing their well-being, and balancing the risks and benefits of participation in evaluation studies. It also explains how to recognize research misconduct.

The evaluator's job is a complex one and includes managing the evaluation project itself. Evaluation project management includes organizing the evaluation team and creating and justifying a budget and a timeline. The chapter provides a job description that lists the skills that program evaluators must have to ensure a successful evaluation. Among these are skills in working independently and in teams, communicating with stakeholders, implementing valid research designs and measurement strategies, analyzing statistical and qualitative data, and supervising project management. Evaluators are also responsible for following a budget, and the chapter gives a

DOI: 10.4324/9781032635071-1

checklist for creating one that will support the team's activities. Keeping to a timeline is extremely important, and the chapter gives an example of a timeline for a four-year evaluation.

A READER'S GUIDE TO CHAPTER 1

What Is Program Evaluation?
  Evaluations of Program Effectiveness
  Evaluations of Program Quality
  Evaluations of Program Value
Evaluation Methods
Selecting Evaluation Questions and Hypotheses
  Providing Evidence of Effectiveness, Quality, and Value
  Designing the Evaluation
  Selecting Participants for the Evaluation
  Collecting Data
  Managing Data and Managing the Evaluation
  Analyzing Data
  Reporting on Effectiveness, Quality, and Value
Who Uses Evaluations?
Baseline Data, Formative Evaluation, and Process Evaluations
  Baseline Data
  Interim Data and Formative Evaluation
  Process or Implementation Evaluation
Summative Evaluation
Qualitative Evaluation
Mixed-Methods Evaluation
Participatory and Collaborative Evaluations: Stakeholder Engagement
Systematic Assessments and True Assessments: What Happens if Traditional Scientific Evaluations Are Not Feasible?
Frameworks and Models for Program Planning and Evaluation
  The PRECEDE-PROCEED Framework
  RE-AIM
  The U.S. Centers for Disease Control's Framework for Planning and Implementing Practical Program Evaluation
Ethics and Program Evaluation
  Evaluations That Need Institutional Review or Ethics Board Approval
  Evaluations That Are Exempt from Ethics Board Approval
  What the IRB Will Review
  Informed Consent
  The Internet and Ethical Evaluations
Research Misconduct
Managing Evaluation Resources
  Program Evaluation Job Description
  Program Evaluation Budgets (and Timelines)
Summary and Transition to the Next Chapter on Evaluation Questions and Evidence of Program Effectiveness, Quality, and Value
Exercises: Chapter 1
References and Suggested Readings
  Suggested Websites
Answers to the Exercises: Chapter 1

WHAT IS PROGRAM EVALUATION?

An evaluation is a systematic assessment of a program's *effectiveness*, *quality*, and *value*. High-quality evaluations are scientific studies that result in unbiased evidence of the program's achievements, impact, and costs. A scientific study answers justified questions about the program by relying on rigorous research design, valid measurements, and appropriate data analytic techniques. An unbiased evaluation is free from systematic errors which are the result of misdirected purpose and flawed study designs and data analysis.

Programs are planned initiatives and interventions to improve the public's quality of life and well-being. They are funded and supported by their stakeholders which include governments, universities, nongovernmental organizations, foundations, trusts, public and private agencies and institutions, and communities of varying sizes and structures. For instance, in a program to evaluate the effectiveness of a UNICEF nutrition program in Kenya, the stakeholders included government ministries and departments (Ministry of Health (MOH), Division of Nutrition and Dietetics; Ministries of Education, Livestock, Agriculture and Fisheries; Labour and Social Protection; Treasury and Planning), implementing partners, County Departments of Health, donor agencies and private sector organizations; UNICEF representatives including decision-makers involved in program planning and design and field teams including zonal officers and nutrition support officers (NSOs); and the communities in which the program was implemented.

Programs and their evaluations are sometimes mandated by law and policy and can be found in almost all fields including education, social welfare, public health, environmental science, medicine, industry, and criminal justice. Stakeholders use evaluation information to understand their program better and to make informed decisions about program improvement, continuation, and funding.

A program may be relatively small (a course in web design for students in two high schools; a new community health center for people over 75 years of age), or relatively large (a nation's universal health plan or a global initiative to eliminate poverty). Programs can take place in differing geographic and political settings, and they vary in their purposes, structures, organization, and constituents.

An effective program achieves positive outcomes and provides measurable benefits to its target population. In an effective program, the benefits are greater than their human and financial costs. A high-quality program meets its stakeholders' needs and is based on sound theory and the best available research evidence. A program's value is measured by its costs and its worth to its stakeholders, the community, and society. Each program evaluation must decide whether it will investigate effectiveness, quality, or value—or all three—a decision sometimes made jointly with stakeholders.

Evaluations take place in many settings, from large urban centers with sophisticated resources and a longstanding dedication to research to relatively small localities that have scant resources and little interest in or knowledge of research or evaluation.

Stakeholders' expectations can vary regardless of where an evaluation takes place, with some people preferring qualitative narratives, while others insist only on statistical data. Some evaluations require evaluators to do a balancing act because they are obligated to fulfill stakeholder expectations (which can differ among themselves), while, at the same time, they must provide evidence-based results that almost always involve statistical data analysis. It is important to acknowledge that the evaluators' responsibility is first and foremost to provide stakeholders with evidence-based information on a program's effectiveness, quality, and value. The surest way to accomplish this objective is through scientific study.

Example 1.1 summarizes three evaluation studies that illustrate what evaluations look like in practice.

Example 1.1 Summaries of Program Evaluations

1. Evaluation of a Healthy Eating Program for Professionals Who Care for Preschoolers (Hardy, King, Kelly, Farrell, & Howlett, 2010)

Background: Early childhood services are a convenient setting for promoting healthy eating and physical activity as a means of preventing overweight and obesity. This evaluation examined the effectiveness of a program to support early childhood professionals in promoting healthy eating and physical activity among children in their care.

Setting and Participants: The evaluation included 15 interventions and 14 control preschools with 430 children whose average age was 4.4 years.

Methods: Preschools were randomly allocated to the intervention or a control program. The evaluators did not know which schools were in each program. They collected data before and after program implementation on children's lunchbox contents; fundamental movement skills (FMS); preschool policies, practices, and staff attitudes; knowledge and confidence related to physical activity; healthy eating; and recreational screen time.

Results: Using statistical methods, the evaluators found that, over time, FMS scores for locomotion and object control, and total FMS scores significantly improved in the intervention group compared with the control group by 3.4, 2.1, and 5.5 points (respectively). The number of FMS sessions per week increased in the intervention group compared with the control group by 1.5. The lunchbox audit showed that children in the intervention group significantly reduced sweetened drinks by 0.13 servings.

Conclusion: The findings suggest that the program effectively improved its targeted weight-related behaviors.

2. Evaluating a Program to Improve the Reading Comprehension of Children at Risk for Language and Literacy Difficulties (Gillam, Vaughan, Roberts, et al., 2023)

This study evaluated the Supporting Knowledge of Language and Literacy (SKILL) program for improving oral narrative comprehension and production among 357 students who were at risk for language and literacy difficulties in Grades 1–4 in 13 schools across seven school districts.

The students were randomly assigned to the SKILL program or a "business as usual" (BAU) control condition. SKILL was provided to small groups of two to four students in 36 thirty-minute lessons across a three-month period. Using a technique of statistical analysis called multilevel modeling, with students "nested" within teachers and teachers "nested" within schools, the evaluators found that immediately after participation, students who were in the SKILL program significantly outperformed students in the BAU condition on measures of oral narrative comprehension and production.

The investigators also found that oral narrative production for the SKILL group remained significantly more advanced five months after the end of study participation. Improvements in oral narration were also found in a measure of written narration both immediately and five months later. Grade level did not alter SKILL's effects on students' oral narration, but it did for reading comprehension, with the program having greater impact among students in Grades 3 and 4.

3. Effect of Internet-Based vs Face-to-Face Cognitive-Behavioral Therapy for Adults with Obsessive-Compulsive Disorder: A Randomized Clinical Trial (Lundström, Flygare, Andersson, et al., 2022)

This study investigated whether therapist-guided and unguided internet-based CBT (ICBT) was noninferior to face-to-face CBT for adults with OCD, conducted a health economic evaluation, and determined whether treatment effects were moderated by source of participant referral.

The study was a single-blinded, noninferiority, randomized clinical trial, with a full health economic evaluation, conducted between, comparing therapist-guided ICBT, unguided ICBT, and individual face-to-face CBT for adults with OCD. The goal of a noninferiority study is to show that the new treatment is not worse than the existing treatment by more than a predetermined amount. Noninferiority studies are often used when there is already an effective treatment available for a particular condition.

Follow-up data was collected up to 12 months after treatment. The study was conducted at two specialist outpatient OCD clinics in Stockholm, Sweden. Participants included a consecutive sample of adults with a primary diagnosis of OCD, either self-referred or referred by a clinician.

The study's primary outcome was the change in OCD symptom severity from baseline to three-month follow-up among the 120 enrolled participants. The investigators found that the mean statistical differences between therapist-guided ICBT and face-to-face CBT at the primary end point were inconclusive. They also found that the difference between unguided ICBT and face-to-face CBT favored face-to-face CBT.

The health economic analysis showed that both guided and unguided ICBT were cost-effective compared with face-to-face CBT. The source of referral did not influence any of the treatment outcomes. The most common adverse events were anxiety (30 participants [25%]), depressive symptoms (20 participants [17%]), and stress (11 participants [9%]).

The study findings did not demonstrate noninferiority among the treatment, but the investigators concluded that therapist-guided ICBT could be a cost-effective alternative to in-clinic CBT for adults with OCD in scenarios where traditional CBT is not readily available; unguided ICBT is probably less effective but could be an alternative when providing remote clinician support is not feasible.

The evaluation summaries in Example 1.1 illustrate that evaluations are complex activities that require multiple skills in research design, statistics, data collection, interpretation, and reporting. Since very few individuals have perfected all these skills, evaluators almost always work in interdisciplinary teams, as is illustrated in Example 1.2.

Example 1.2 Program Evaluation is Interdisciplinary

- A four-year evaluation of a new workplace literacy program was conducted by a team composed of two professional evaluators, a survey researcher, a statistician, and two instructors. The evaluation team also consulted an economist and an expert in information science.
- A three-year evaluation of a 35-project program to improve access to and use of social services for low-income women relied on two professional evaluators, a social worker, an epidemiologist, a nurse practitioner, an economist, and a communications specialist to help report results to participating women.
- An evaluation of a program using nurses to screen community-dwelling elderly individuals for hypertension, vision, and hearing disorders relied on a nurse, a nurse practitioner, a statistician, and a professional evaluator.

Evaluations of Program Effectiveness

An effective program provides measurable and enduring benefits, and the benefits are greater than their human and financial costs. Effectiveness evaluations provide answers to questions like:

- Did the program achieve its objectives and planned outcomes for all participants?
- Which participants achieved the most benefit?
- Did the benefits last over time?
- Were there any unanticipated outcomes or harm due to participation?
- Were any components of the program more beneficial than others?
- Which components of the program need improvement?

Not all programs are effective even if they are funded well and are enthusiastically supported by stakeholders. Because of this, evaluators must conduct evaluations that adhere closely to the scientific method because only then can they provide unbiased, objective evidence to support their findings. Negative findings are arguably as important as positive findings because they, too, provide crucial information for informed decision-making.

Evaluations of Program Quality

High-quality programs meet their users' needs and are based on accepted theories of human behavior and the best available research evidence. They have sufficient funding to ensure that their objectives are achieved and have strong leadership, trained staff, and a supportive environment.

Commonly asked questions about program quality include:

- Has the program been studied systematically before implementation so that its risks and benefits are predictable?
- Is the program grounded in theory or supported by the best available research?
- Does the program provide a safe, healthy, and nurturing environment for all participants?
- Is the infrastructure well developed, and is the fiscal management sound?
- How well does the program develop and nurture positive relationships among staff, participants, and communities?
- Does the program recruit, hire, and train a diverse staff who value each participant and can deliver services as planned at the highest level?
- Does the program have a coherent mission and a plan for increasing capacity so that the program is sustained or continues to grow?
- Is a system in place for measuring outcomes and using that information for program planning, improvement, and evaluation?
- Are resources appropriately allocated so that each component of the program and its evaluation are likely to produce unbiased and timely information?

Evaluations of Program Value

Value is defined as the importance, worth, or usefulness of something. The term value is subjective, and the whole enterprise of program evaluation is based on using scientific methods to minimize the subjectivity—bias—that can consume the process of analyzing or judging a program.

One interpretation of value is the costs of a program costs and the relationship of costs to effectiveness and benefit. Program costs include any risks or problems that adversely affect program participants. For instance, program participants in a group therapy program may feel embarrassed about revealing personal information, or they may become unexpectedly ill from the treatment being evaluated. Program costs also include the financial costs of facilities, staff, and equipment.

Typical questions about program costs include:

- If two programs achieve similar outcomes, which one is less costly?
- For each euro, dollar, or pound spent, how much is saved on future use of services?

Typical evaluation questions about program value include:

- What are the costs and risks of program participation?
- Do the program's benefits outweigh its costs?
- Does the program meet a need that no other service can or does provide?
- Does the program provide the most improvement and benefits possible with its available resources?

EVALUATION METHODS

Program evaluation relies on the scientific method to gather unbiased evidence to support its findings. The scientific method involves identifying justifiable questions and hypotheses; setting standards for acceptable evidence of effectiveness, quality, or value; designing a rigorous study; collecting valid data to answer the question; analyzing the data; and reporting results. Example 1.3 illustrates the use of the scientific method in planning an evaluation of a mindfulness program for people with chronic pain.

Example 1.3 Using the Scientific Method to Plan an Evaluation of a Mindfulness Program

Question: Can a mindfulness program improve the mental health of people with chronic pain?

Justification: There is growing evidence that mindfulness can be an effective intervention for a variety of mental health conditions, including anxiety and depression. Mindfulness is the practice of paying attention to the present moment without judgment. It can be practiced through meditation, yoga, or other activities.

Null hypothesis: The experiment and control participants will not differ in their mental health after the experimental program is completed.

Evidence of effectiveness: For the primary outcome, a statistical difference in depression scores from baseline to eight weeks, favoring the experimental group over the control. Secondary outcomes will include favorable statistically observed changes in anxiety scores, pain scores, and quality-of-life scores. If statistical differences are observed, the null hypothesis will be rejected.

Evaluation study design: People with chronic pain will be identified by their clinicians and randomly assigned either to a mindfulness program group or to a control group. The mindfulness program group will receive weekly mindfulness training for eight weeks. The control group will not receive any intervention.

Data collection measures: Scores on validated measures of depression, anxiety, pain, and quality of life will be administered at baseline and immediately after program conclusion at eight weeks.

Data analysis: Statistical tests for differences in scores on each measure between the two groups.

Conclusions: If the results of the study are positive and favor the experimental group, they will constitute evidence that mindfulness can be an effective intervention for improving the mental health of people with chronic pain. This can lead to the development of new mindfulness-based interventions for people with chronic pain.

Reporting: The evaluation team will report the results of their study at the annual meeting of the Mental Health Institute (which provided the funds for the evaluation) and at professional conferences attended by mental health providers.

SELECTING EVALUATION QUESTIONS AND HYPOTHESES

Evaluations begin by identifying questions or hypotheses that will produce the information that stakeholders need to make decisions about their program. Typical generic evaluation questions and hypotheses include:

*   **Question:** Did the program achieve its goals and objectives?
    Hypothesis: When compared to a similar program, program A will achieve significantly more goals and objectives than Program B.

- **Question:** Which program characteristics (theoretical foundation, use of technology, funding) are most likely responsible for the best and worst outcomes?
  Hypothesis: The online course will achieve significantly better results than the traditional course.
- **Question:** For which individuals or groups was the program most effective?
  Hypothesis: Boys and girls will achieve the same reading levels.
- **Question:** How applicable are the program's objectives and activities to other participants in other settings?
  Hypothesis: Participants in other schools will do as well as participants in the local school.
- **Question**: How enduring were the program's outcomes?
  Hypothesis: Participants will maintain their gains over a five-year period after the program's conclusion.
- **Question:** What are the relationships between the costs of the program and its outcomes?
  Hypothesis: For every $10 spent, there will be at least one reading level improvement.
- **Question:** To what extent did social, political, and financial support influence the program's outcomes and acceptability?
  Hypothesis: Local support is associated with greater program satisfaction.
- **Question:** Is the program cost-effective?
  Hypothesis: New Program A and Old Program B achieve similar outcomes, but Program A costs less to implement.
- **Question:** Were there any unanticipated outcomes (beneficial as well as harmful)?

This is a research question. No hypothesis is associated with it because the evaluators have no basis for stating one. They do not have a theory or any research evidence to support assumptions about outcomes.

Some evaluations answer just a few questions or test just a few hypotheses, while others answer many questions and test numerous hypotheses. The number will depend upon the users' needs and the evaluation's resources.

Providing Evidence of Effectiveness, Quality, and Value

The evidence used in an evaluation consists of the facts and observations that convince users that the program's benefits outweigh its risks and costs. Convincing evidence may come from personal preference, professional experience, or statistical tests. Consider each of the following seven possible types of evidence for a program whose objective is "to improve children's dietary and other health habits":

1. Testimony from children in the program (and from their parents and teachers) that their habits have improved.
2. The evaluator's observations of improved health habits (through studies of children's choices of snacks during and between meals).
3. Proof of children's improved health status found in physical examinations by a nurse practitioner or a physician.
4. The evaluator's finding of statistically significant differences in habits and in health status between children who are in the program compared with children who are not. Children in the program do significantly better.
5. The evaluator's finding of statistically significant and sustained differences in habits and in health status between children who are in the program compared with children who are not. Children in the program continue to do significantly better over a two-year period.
6. Statistical and qualitative evidence that Program A achieves the same aims as Program B and that it is less costly.

7. Qualitative and statistical evidence that the program is based on a validated model of children's health behavior, and that statistically significantly more children enjoyed their participation in it than did children in two other programs with similar objectives.

Which of these seven possibilities is the "best" evidence of the program's effectiveness, quality, and value? The evaluator's challenge in answering this question is to find out which of them is convincing to the evaluation's users and funding agencies and can be obtained with the available resources. For instance, evaluators are unlikely to be able to provide data on whether program effects last for two years (possibility #5), if the evaluation only has funds for a one-year study.

Many evaluators consult and form partnerships with users and funders to ensure that the evidence they provide is appropriate and likely to meet expectations. Evaluators find that working with clients typically creates mutual respect, promotes client cooperation with data collection during the evaluation's implementation, and improves the usefulness of the results.

Designing the Evaluation

An evaluation's design is its structure. Evaluators do their best to design a project so that any program benefits the evaluators find are unbiased and not influenced by expectation or preference. A standard evaluation design includes comparing the participants in a new program with participants in an alternative program. The comparison can occur once or several times. For example, suppose five universities plan to participate in an evaluation of a new program to teach the basic principles of program evaluation to Education Corps trainees. In designing the study, the evaluator must answer questions like these:

- Which program is a fair comparison to the "new" one? Evaluators sometimes compare the new program to an already existing one with similar characteristics, or they compare the new program to "usual practice." If the resources are available, they may compare the new program to an already existing program and to usual practice. Another option is to compare two versions of the new program and usual practice. For instance, a crime prevention program for teens may compare a smartphone app with peer counseling [version 1], the same app without the counseling [version 2], and the school's usual monthly webinar [usual practice].
- Which criteria are appropriate for including institutions? (Size? Resources? Location?)
- Which criteria are appropriate for excluding institutions? (Unwillingness to implement the program as planned? Lack of staff commitment to the evaluation?)
- What should I measure? Which beliefs, preferences, and behaviors?
- When should I measure? (Before and after program participation? How long after program participation?)

Selecting Participants for the Evaluation

Suppose you are asked to evaluate a program to provide school-based mental health services to children who have witnessed or have been victims of violence in their communities. Here are some questions you need to ask:

- Who should be included in the evaluation? (How old should the children be? How much exposure to violence should eligible children have?)
- Who should be excluded? (Should children be excluded if, in the opinion of the mental health clinician, they are probably too disruptive to participate in the program's required group therapy sessions?)

- How many children should be included? (How many children should be studied so that the evaluation has enough to detect changes in children's behavior if the program is effective?)

Collecting Data

Conclusions about a program's effectiveness, quality, and value come from the data an evaluator collects to answer questions and test hypotheses. Data collection includes:

- identifying the variables (individual knowledge, attitudes, or behaviors; community practices; social policies) that are the program's target outcomes
- identifying the characteristics of the participants who will be affected by the program (men between the ages of 45 and 54, rural and urban communities)
- selecting, adapting, or creating measures of the variables (knowledge tests, direct observations of behavior; analysis of legal documents)
- demonstrating the reliability (consistency) and validity (accuracy) of the measures
- administering the measures
- analyzing and interpreting the results.

Some common measures or sources of evaluation data are:

- literature reviews
- existing databases, such as those maintained by governments, hospitals, and schools
- self-administered questionnaires (including in-person, mailed, and online surveys)
- interviews (in person and on the phone)
- achievement tests
- observations in person or by reviewing audio or video formats
- physical examinations
- hypothetical vignettes or case studies.

Managing Data and Managing the Evaluation

The term *data management* refers to what evaluators do with data from the moment it is collected until it is ready to be shared with other evaluators, researchers, program developers and participants, policy experts, and funding agencies. *Managing the evaluation* means organizing an evaluation team and preparing and adhering to a realistic budget and timeline.

Data management incorporates many tasks and requires statistical and database management expertise. The tasks include selecting a statistical software platform, planning the data analysis, and overseeing or doing data entry and data analysis. A singularly important evaluation data management responsibility is the documentation of all analytic activities including a detailed report on how the variables in each evaluation question or hypothesis were defined and coded, why each analytic method was selected to answer the question or test the hypothesis, and how to use the database in other evaluations or to replicate the current one.

Program evaluators are often responsible for managing some or all of the evaluation's activities and resources. Program evaluation management includes hiring personnel and preparing budgets and timelines. Program evaluations can be very large (such as the five-year evaluation of a worldwide initiative to provide elementary school education to children in rural areas) or relatively small (such as the one-year evaluation of a new reading program in one school). Thus, the staffing and resources will differ according to the size and scope of the evaluation, and evaluators must be prepared to ensure that the evaluation team has the skills and the financial resources to successfully complete all activities on time.

A job description for a program evaluator will ask for people who have a combination of skills including expertise in program evaluation principles, research design, data collection and statistical analysis, communication, program content knowledge, and team coordination. Preparing evaluation budgets and timelines involves learning about personnel costs, the level of staff effort and time needed to accomplish each task and preparing a realistic timeline.

Analyzing Data

Data analysis consists of the descriptive (qualitative) and statistical (quantitative) methods used to summarize information about a program's effectiveness, quality, and value. The choice of which method of analysis to use is dependent on several considerations.

- The characteristics of the evaluation question or hypothesis and evidence of effectiveness, quality, and value. (Do the questions ask about differences over time among groups or about associations between program characteristics and benefits? If the questions ask about differences, then a statistical method that tests for differences is needed. If the questions ask about associations, then different statistical methods are probably warranted.)
- How the variables are expressed statistically: categorically ("did or did not pass the test"); ordinally (Stage I, II, or III of a disease; ratings on a scale ranging from 1 to 5); or numerically (average scores on a mathematics test).
- How the variables are expressed qualitatively (themes from an analysis of a focus group).
- The reliability and validity of the data.

Reporting on Effectiveness, Quality, and Value

An evaluation report describes, justifies, and explains the purposes of the evaluation, the program, the setting, and the methods that are used to arrive at unbiased conclusions about effectiveness, quality, and value. The methods include descriptions and explanations of the evaluation questions and evidence selection processes, the research design, sampling strategy, data collection, and data analysis. The report also states the results and arrives at conclusions about program effectiveness, quality, and value based on the evidence. Many journals also require proof that the evaluation respected and protected participants from risk. This is done by asking for the evaluator to state that the evaluation received a formal review by an ethics board.

Evaluation reports may be oral (slide presentations in person or online), or printed (in professional journals, newspapers, or online).

You can find evaluation reports and research in their entirety online. There are hundreds of databases, online libraries, and open access journals that contain evaluation studies. Some are free like PubMed (https://pubmed.ncbi.nlm.nih.gov) and the Educational Resources Information Center or ERIC (https://eric.ed.gov), while others require paid membership (PsycInfo, Web of Science).

WHO USES EVALUATIONS?

At least eight different stakeholder groups use the information that results from program evaluations:

1. Government agencies.
2. Program developers (a director of a community health clinic, a curriculum committee, or a nursing school's curriculum committee).

3. Communities (geographically intact areas, such as a city's "skid row"; people with a share health-related problem, such as HIV/AIDS).
4. Policy makers (elected officials; the school board).
5. Program funding agencies (philanthropic foundations or trusts and the various agencies of the U.S. National Institutes of Health or the UK National Health Service).
6. Students, researchers, and other evaluators (in schools and universities, government agencies, businesses, and public agencies).
7. Individuals interested in new programs.
8. Program/evaluation participants.

BASELINE DATA, FORMATIVE EVALUATION, AND PROCESS EVALUATIONS

The need for a program is demonstrated when there is a gap between what individuals or communities need and their current services. Baseline data is collected to document program participants' status before they begin the program. Interim data, which is collected during the program, provide preliminary information on the program's implementation and effects. This interim data is used to evaluate the program while in its formative stage.

Baseline Data

Baseline data is collected before the start of the program to describe the characteristics of participants (e.g., their social, educational, health status and demographic features, such as age), information that is important later when the evaluator is interpreting the effects of the program on its participants.

Example 1.4 illustrates some of the reasons program evaluators collect baseline data.

Example 1.4 Baseline Data and Program Evaluation

The Agency for Drug and Alcohol Misuse has published extensive guidelines for identifying and counseling adolescents whose alcohol use is interfering with their everyday activities, such as attendance at school. An evaluation of the guidelines' effectiveness is being conducted nationwide. Before the evaluators begin the formal evaluation process, they collect baseline data on the extent to which health care professionals in different settings (e.g., schools and community clinics) already follow the practices recommended by the guidelines, the prevalence of alcohol misuse among adolescents in the communities of interest, and the number of adolescents that are likely to use services in the evaluation's proposed duration of three years.

Interim Data and Formative Evaluation

In a formative evaluation, data is collected after the start of a program, but before its conclusion—for example, 12 months after the beginning of a three-year intervention.
An evaluator collects interim data to describe the progress of the program while it is still developing or "forming." Formative evaluation data is mainly useful to program developers and funding agencies. Program developers and funders may want to know if a new program is feasible as is, or if it needs to be changed. A feasible program is one that can be implemented according to plan and is likely to be beneficial.

Data from formative evaluations is always preliminary and requires cautious interpretation. Example 1.5 illustrates why evaluators need to take care in interpreting formative findings.

Example 1.5 Formative Evaluation and Interim Data: Proceed with Caution

In a three-year study of access to prenatal care, the results of a 14-month formative evaluation found that three of six community clinics had opened on schedule and were providing services to needy women exactly as planned. Preliminary data also revealed that 200 women had been served in the clinics, and that the proportion of babies born weighing less than 2,500 grams (5.5 pounds) was 4%, well below the state's average of 6%. The evaluators concluded that progress was being made toward improving access to prenatal care. After three years, however, the evaluation results were quite different. The remaining three scheduled clinics had never opened, and one of the original three clinics had closed. Many fewer women were served than had been anticipated, and the proportion of low-birthweight babies was 6.6%.

As this example shows, data from a formative evaluation can be misleading. Good interim results may be exhilarating, but poor ones can adversely affect staff morale. With programs of relatively short duration—say, two years or less—the collection of interim data is expensive and probably not very useful. Consider the evaluation described in Example 1.6.

Example 1.6 Questions Asked in a Formative Evaluation of a Program for Critically Ill Children

Many experts agree that the emergency medical services needed by critically ill and injured children differ in important ways from those needed by adults. As a result, several health regions have attempted to reorganize their emergency services to provide better care to children. One region commissioned a three-year evaluation of its program. It was specifically concerned with the characteristics and effectiveness of a soon-to-be-implemented intervention to prevent transfers from adult inpatient or intensive care units and to maximize quality of care for children with cardiopulmonary arrest in hospital emergency departments and intensive care units.

In planning the evaluation, the evaluators decided to check a sample of medical records in 15 of the state's 56 counties to see whether sufficient information was available for them to use the records as a main source of data. Also, the evaluators planned to release preliminary findings after 12 months, which involved reviews of records as well as interviews with physicians, hospital administrators, paramedics, and patients' families. An expert's review of the evaluation's design raised these questions for the evaluators:

1. Does the description of this evaluation as a "three-year evaluation" mean that there will be three years of data collection, or does it mean that the three years include evaluation planning, implementation, and reporting as well as data collection? Assume interim data is promised in a year. Can you develop and validate medical record review forms in time to collect enough information to present meaningful findings?
2. Can you develop, validate, and administer the survey forms in the time available?
3. To what extent will the interim and preliminary analyses answer the same or similar questions? If they are very different, will you have sufficient time and money to effectively conduct both?
4. Will a written or oral interim report be required? How long will that take to prepare?

Some program evaluations are divided into two phases. In Phase 1, the evaluation is designed to focus on feasibility and improvement, and in Phase 2, it focuses on effectiveness, cost, and value. Some funding agencies prefer to have Phase 1 done internally by the participating schools or clinics, and Phase 2 done externally by independent, preferably external evaluation consultants. External evaluations are presumed to be more objective and less inclined to bias than internal evaluations.

Process or Implementation Evaluations

A process evaluation, which is sometimes called an implementation evaluation, is concerned with the extent to which planned program and evaluation activities are implemented, and its findings may be reported at any time during the evaluation's course. Process evaluations provide information on what is being done in the name of the program. Programs are not always implemented according to plan for many reasons including improper staff training, competing priorities, and unforeseen circumstances. Example 1.7 discusses an evaluation of three programs to increase the rates at which women returned to follow up on an abnormal test result. The process evaluation concluded that implementation of the three programs was less than perfect, and thus introduced a bias into the results of the effectiveness evaluation.

Example 1.7 Process or Implementation Evaluation

During a two-year evaluation, all women were to be surveyed at least once regarding whether they received their assigned program as planned and the extent to which they understood its purposes and adhered to its requirements. Telephone interviews after 18 months revealed that 74 of 100 women (74%) who were in the in-person video-based program had seen the entire 25-minute presentation and were reminded to come back for another follow-up test, while only 70 of 111 (63%) women in the online video-based program were reminded, and just 32 of 101 (about 32%) of the participatory video conference program were reminded. The fact that only one-third of participants in the in-person video group received the program as planned helped to explain its apparent failure to achieve positive results when compared with the other two groups.

SUMMATIVE EVALUATION

Summative evaluations are historical studies that are compiled after the program has been in existence for a while (say, two years), or all program activities have officially ceased. These evaluations sum up and qualitatively assess the program's development and achievements.

Summative evaluations are descriptive rather than experimental studies. Evaluation funding agencies sometimes request these evaluations because summative reports may contain details on how many people the program served, how the staff was trained, how barriers to implementation were overcome, and if participants were satisfied and likely to benefit. Summative evaluations often provide a thorough explanation of how the program was developed and the social and political context in which the program and its evaluation were conducted.

QUALITATIVE EVALUATION

Qualitative evaluations collect data through interviews, direct observations, and review of written documents (e.g., private diaries kept for the evaluation). The aim of these evaluations is to provide personalized information on the dynamics of a program and on participants' perceptions of the program's outcomes and impact.

Qualitative evaluation is useful for examining programs where the goals are in the process of being defined, and for testing out the workability of evaluation methods. Because they are personalized, qualitative methods may add emotion and depth to statistical findings.

Qualitative methods are employed in program evaluations to complement the usual sources of data (such as standardized surveys, database reviews, and achievement tests). Example 1.8 illustrates four uses of qualitative methods in program evaluation.

Example 1.8 Uses of Qualitative Methods in Program Evaluation

1. To evaluate the effectiveness of a campaign to get heroin addicts to clean their needles with bleach, the evaluators spend time in a heroin "shooting gallery." They do not have formal observation measures, although they do take notes. The evaluators discuss what they have seen, and although needles are being cleaned, they agree that the addicts use a common dish to rinse needles and dilute the drug before shooting. The evaluators recommend that the community's program should be altered to consider the dangers of this practice.
2. To evaluate the quality and effectiveness of an education counseling program for mentally ill adults, the evaluation team lives for three months in each of five different residential communities. After taping more than 250 counseling sessions, the evaluators examine the tape to determine if certain counseling approaches were used consistently. They conclude that the quality of the counseling varies greatly both within and among the communities, which helps to explain the overall program's inconsistent results.
3. To evaluate the impact of a school-based health program for homeless children, the evaluators teach a cohort of children to keep diaries over a three-year period. The evaluation finds that children in the program are much more willing to attend to the dangers of smoking and other drug use than are children in schools without the program. The evaluators do an analysis of the content of the children's diaries. They find that children in the program are especially pleased to participate. The evaluators conclude that the children's enjoyment may be related to the program's positive outcomes.
4. An evaluation of the impact on the province of a program to improve access to and use of prenatal care services asks "opinion leaders" to give their views. These people are known in the province to have expertise in providing, financing, and evaluating prenatal care. The interviewers encourage the leaders to raise any issues of concern. The leaders share their belief that any improvements in prenatal care are probably due to medical advances rather than to enhanced access to services. After the interviews are completed, the evaluators conclude that major barriers to access and use continue to exist even though statistical registries reveal a decline in infant mortality rates for some groups of women.

In the first evaluation in Example 1.8, the evaluators are observers at the heroin shooting gallery. They rely on their observations and notes to come to agreement on their recommendations. In the second illustration, the evaluators tape the sessions and then interpret the results. The interpretations come after the data is collected; the evaluators make no effort to state evaluation questions in advance of data collection. In the third illustration, diaries are used as a qualitative tool, allowing participants to say how they feel in their own words. In the fourth illustration in Example 1.8, experts are invited to give their own views; the evaluators make little attempt to require the opinion leaders to adhere to certain topics.

MIXED-METHODS EVALUATION

Mixed methods are a type of research in which qualitative data and quantitative or statistical data are combined within a single study. Example 1.9 outlines at least three reasons for mixing methods: to better understand experimental study results, to incorporate user perspectives into program development, and to answer differing research questions within the same study.

Example 1.9 Reasons for Mixed-Methods Evaluations

1. Mixed Methods Incorporate User Perspectives into Program Development

The study's main purpose was to develop online education to improve people's use of web-based health information. The investigators convened five focus groups and conducted in-depth interviews with 15 people to identify preferences for learning [user perspectives]. They asked participants questions about the value of audio and video presentations. Using the information from the groups and interviews, the investigators developed an online education tutorial and observed its usability in a small sample. Once they had evidence that the education was ready for use in the general population, they evaluated its effectiveness by using statistical methods to compare the knowledge, self-efficacy, and internet use among two groups. Group 1 was assigned to use the newly created online tutorial, and Group 2 was given a printed checklist containing tips for reliable online health information searches.

2. Mixed Methods Answer Different Research Questions in the Same Study (Marczinski & Stamates, 2013)

The investigators aimed to find out if alcohol consumed with an artificially sweetened mixer (diet soft drink) results in higher breath alcohol concentrations (BrACs) compared with the same amount of alcohol consumed with a similar beverage containing sugar [Research Question 1]. They also intended to determine if individuals are aware of the differences [Research Question 2]. BrACs were recorded, as were self-reported ratings of subjective intoxication, fatigue, impairment, and willingness to drive. Performance was assessed using a signaled go/no-go reaction time task. Based on the results, the investigators found that mixing alcohol with a diet soft drink results in elevated BrACs, as compared with the same amount of alcohol mixed with a sugar-sweetened beverage. Individuals are unaware of these differences, a factor that may increase the safety risks associated with drinking alcohol.

3. Mixed Methods Help Evaluators Better Understand Experimental Results

The investigators found that experimental program participants reported significantly more discomfort with study participation than did control program participants. This finding surprised the evaluation team. To help them understand the findings, the team conducted interviews with each of the experimental program participants and asked them about the causes of their discomfort.

PARTICIPATORY AND COLLABORATIVE EVALUATIONS: STAKEHOLDER ENGAGEMENT

A *participatory or collaborative evaluation* invites *stakeholders* to actively join in directing and monitoring some or all evaluation's activities. Stakeholders are representatives of the communities, organizations, and institutions that are directly affected by the evaluation or fund it. Stakeholder participation or collaboration results in useful and authentic evaluations for four reasons:

1. Stakeholder participation helps to improve the quality and validity of evaluation by giving it a basis in local knowledge, culture, and history. In participatory evaluations, public concerns are viewed ecologically—that is, within their political and social context as well as within their clinical or institutional setting.
2. Including the expertise of stakeholders enhances the relevance of the evaluation's purpose and questions, the quality and quantity of data gathered, and the use of the data. Stakeholders as well as evaluators "own" the data and therefore want to see the data used.

3. Participatory evaluation projects can assist in providing stakeholders with resources and possible employment opportunities. For example, community members can help evaluators in translating surveys and in conducting interviews.
4. Participatory evaluations can lead to improvements in the health and well-being of communities by studying and addressing important community needs and increasing community members' power and control over the evaluation process. Stakeholders can keep the evaluators on track, preventing them from taking an approach that is too abstract or perhaps conversely too focused on efficiency.

Example 1.10 provides illustrations of participatory evaluation in action.

Example 1.10 Participatory Evaluations in Action

1. An evaluation of a cancer control program involves the community in all phases of the project, from the development of the grant proposal through to interpretation of the data. The purpose of the project is to evaluate the effectiveness of a culturally appropriate intervention as a means of increasing breast and cervical cancer screening practice among the community's women. The results show a community-wide impact on cancer-related knowledge, attitudes, and behaviors; increased research capabilities; and improvements to the health systems and services available to the community.
2. A mental health intervention is designed to diminish symptoms of depression in urban schoolchildren who have witnessed or participated in community violence. A group of parents assists the evaluators in developing evaluation questions, translating some of the surveys from English into Spanish and Russian, and collecting data from other parents. They also review the evaluation's findings and comment on them. The comments are incorporated into the final report of the intervention's effectiveness.
3. The directors of a health care clinic, interested in improving patient education, intend to organize a series of staff seminars and then evaluate whether patient education improves after all staff have attended the seminars. As part of the evaluation, the evaluation team convenes a series of four noon meetings with clinic staff to identify the nature and extent of current problems in the clinic's education for patients and to examine alternative solutions. The clinic staff agrees to form a committee to work with the evaluators and decide on evidence of effectiveness for the seminars and patient education. The staff also agrees to advise the evaluators on questions to ask patients about their experiences at the clinic and to review and comment on the report of the evaluation's findings.

In the first illustration in Example 1.10, members of the community are actively included in all phases of the evaluation study, including the writing of the proposal for funding and the interpretation of the data. In the second instance, parents work with the evaluators on many activities, including the formulation of evaluation questions, data collection, and reporting. They are not necessarily involved in designing the evaluation (determining which children are eligible for participation and the characteristics of the control or comparative intervention) or in the data analysis. The third illustration is a participatory evaluation because the staff and evaluators work together to decide on evidence of effectiveness, identify appropriate questions to ask patients about their experiences, and review the evaluation report.

Participatory evaluators must be skilled in working with diverse groups of individuals. They must learn how to lead meetings, encourage consensus, and inform participants about the objectives and purposes of evaluation studies in general and their own evaluations in particular. At the same time, participatory evaluators must lead the process of collecting unbiased data and interpreting those data objectively.

Not all programs—no matter how well intentioned—are effective, and even those that have positive effects may not be cost-effective, and so the participatory evaluator must be prepared to be the bearer of bad news. Participatory evaluations themselves also tend to be extremely costly because they are labor-intensive: They require individuals from the evaluation team and the community to spend time agreeing on evidence of effectiveness, quality, and value, and spend time assisting with technical activities, including research design, data collection, and report writing.

SYSTEMATIC ASSESSMENTS AND TRUE EXPERIMENTS: WHAT HAPPENS IF TRADITIONAL SCIENTIFIC EVALUATIONS ARE NOT FEASIBLE?

Program evaluation is defined as a systematic assessment of a program's effectiveness, quality, and value. The highest-quality evaluations are scientific studies that result in unbiased evidence of the program's achievements, impact, and costs. But what should evaluators do in circumstances in which the program's size, location, or evaluation budget are not conducive to a true experiment? Example 1.11 illustrates a setting in which a true experiment would not have been realistic.

Example 1.11 Settings in Which Traditional Scientific Evaluations Are Not Feasible (Codjia, Kutondo, Kamudoni, et al., 2022)

Mid-Term Evaluation of Maternal and Child Nutrition Programme in Kenya. UNICEF's Maternal and Child Nutrition Programme is a four-year (2018–2022) resilience-building, multi-sectoral program focused on pregnant and lactating women, mothers of children under five years, and children under five years. The objective of the mid-term evaluation was to establish the relevance, effectiveness, efficiency, and sustainability of the program, whose target population consisted of the most marginalized communities in the country.

The evaluation used a non-experimental concurrent mixed-method approach. Qualitative information was gathered through 29 key informant interviews and 18 focus group discussions (six focus groups per population group: women of reproductive age, adolescent girls, and men). Quantitative data was obtained through reviews of secondary data from program reports, budgets, and project outputs.

The evaluation in Example 1.11 deals with a large nationwide program, and the logistics and costs of a true experiment would have been infeasible. The study is, however, systematic and transparent, and the evaluators carefully describe the study's limitations, facilitating its findings' usefulness.

When evaluators cannot realistically conduct traditional experiments, they can still systematically assess programs by using other methods such as case studies, qualitative research, and mixed-methods research.

A case study is an in-depth examination of a single program or group of participants. Case studies can be useful for understanding the context in which a program operated and how the program was planned and implemented.

Qualitative research, which involves collecting data through interviews, focus groups, and other methods that allow for in-depth exploration of people's experiences, can be useful for understanding how participants feel about their participation, and why they feel that way. It can also uncover suggestions for improving the program and the evaluation.

Mixed-methods research combines quantitative and qualitative data collection methods. To get the most reliable information possible, regardless of the research type they use, evaluators should use a variety of data collection methods rather than just one, and the measures they use should be valid ones.

Evaluators who use alternatives to traditional true experiments must be particularly transparent about their study's limitations. They must avoid making causal claims about the program's effectiveness, quality, or value. Instead, they should focus on describing the program's activities and on compiling evidence of the factors that may have contributed to the program's success or failure. The evidence should be decided together with community and funder stakeholders to ensure usefulness and credibility.

The evaluation's studied outcomes should focus on very specific measurable objectives (to provide everyday access to clean water to 50 families within the next 12 months). In some situations, it can be appropriate to do a scientific evaluation of a portion of the program in a few communities or among a subset of the larger population.

FRAMEWORKS AND MODELS FOR PROGRAM PLANNING AND EVALUATION

The PRECEDE-PROCEED Framework

Evaluation frameworks provide guidance for program planners and evaluators, helping ensure that the evaluation's overall design considers the origins and contexts of the program about to be evaluated. Frameworks are particularly useful if the evaluators are also part of the program planning process because they focus attention on the setting and resources that are most likely to facilitate efficient program implementation. One commonly used framework is the PRECEDE-PROCEED Framework.

The acronym PRECEDE stands for predisposing, reinforcing, and enabling constructs in education/environmental diagnosis and evaluation. The acronym PROCEED stands for policy, regulatory, and organizational constructs in educational and environmental development. Although developed to study how programs influence changes in health behavior, PRECEDE-PROCEED is being used increasingly in the fields or disciplines of education and psychology and in many community-based programs.

The PRECEDE-PROCEED MODEL is applied in nine phases:

1. **Social assessment** to determine perceptions of people's needs and quality of life. For instance, evaluators use focus groups with parents, students, and teachers to find out how to improve attendance at after school programs.
2. **Epidemiological assessment** to identify the problems that are most important in the community. For instance, evaluators conduct interviews with providers at local clinics to find out why neighborhood children visit the clinics; evaluators review county records to study inoculation rates; program planners conduct interviews with children and families to learn more about their culture, family history, and lifestyle.
3. **Educational and ecological assessment** to identify the factors that might be needed to foster changes in behaviors. These may include assessments of knowledge, beliefs, and self-efficacy (referred to as predisposing factors); social support (reinforcing factors); and programs and services necessary for good outcomes to be realized (enabling factors).
4. **Administrative and policy assessment and intervention alignment** to review policies and resources that facilitate or hinder program implementation.
5–9. **Implementation and evaluation of process, impact, and outcomes.** Using the assessments as a guide, program developers implement programs, and evaluators study the programs' activities and immediate and long-term outcomes.

RE-AIM

The acronym RE-AIM stands for reach, efficacy (or effectiveness), adoption, implementation, and maintenance. *Reach* refers to the percentage of potential participants who are exposed to a program and how representative they are of others who might benefit from it. *Efficacy* or *effectiveness* refers to the intended and unintended effects of a program. *Adoption* includes attention to the participation rate of eligible subjects and how well the setting and the people who deliver the program reflect future participants. *Implementation* denotes the extent to which various components of the program are delivered as intended. *Maintenance* is related to two questions: What are the program's long-term effects? To what extent is the program continued after the completion of the evaluation?

The U.S. Centers for Disease Control's Framework for Planning and Implementing Practical Program Evaluation

Figure 1.1 illustrates the framework for planning and implementing "practical" program evaluation recommended by the U.S. Centers for Disease Control and Prevention (CDC). There are six steps for accomplishing the evaluation and four standards for assessing the evaluation: accuracy, utility, feasibility, and propriety. The six steps involve engaging stakeholders, describing the program, focusing the evaluation design, gathering credible evidence justifying conclusions, and ensuring use learned. An effective evaluation serves the information needs of intended users (utility), is realistic (feasibility), reveals technically accurate information (accuracy), and is conducted legally, ethically, and with regard for those involved and affected (propriety).

The three frameworks described above share several important features. First, they are all frameworks, and not models. Their purpose is to provide guidance in program planning and evaluation. Models "predict" behavior or outcomes and are based on theoretical expectations or empirical evidence gained through experience and experiment. Frameworks leave the theories and methods of implementation to the evaluator.

These three frameworks are all-inclusive. PRECEDE-PROCEED, for example, contains a comprehensive set of factors that should be considered in program planning and evaluation. It is unlikely, however, that evaluators will ever find themselves involved in all aspects of program development and evaluation as characterized in this framework. In most cases, evaluators are

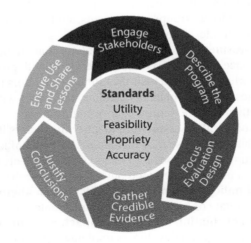

Figure 1.1 The U.S. Centers for Disease Control and Prevention's Framework for Program Evaluation

called in to appraise the effectiveness of existing programs. No one really expects an individual evaluator to be an expert in the planning process or in the development of a program which almost always involves subject-matter knowledge. The evaluator's primary domain is collecting and interpreting unbiased data on the implementation of the program and investigating its effectiveness, quality, and value.

Frameworks, such as PRECEDE-PROCEED, RE-AIM, and the CDC's approach to practical evaluation are useful in encouraging evaluators to pay attention to the origins and development of the programs they examine (even if the evaluator had little to do with establishing the need for the programs or with their implementation). Any knowledge an evaluator gains may help in designing realistic and relevant evaluation studies.

The CDC's framework is different from PRECEDE-PROCEED and RE-AIM in that it incorporates standards that include propriety. Propriety refers to the legal and ethical considerations involved in evaluation research. Except for very small, local studies, most evaluation studies are now required by law and institutional practice to demonstrate their ethical nature in writing, specifying how they will show respect for their participants and protect participants' privacy.

ETHICS AND PROGRAM EVALUATION

Program evaluations almost always involve people as research participants. There are exceptions—for example, when institutions are compared to evaluate the effectiveness of different governance systems in improving efficiency, or when businesses promote programs to improve the quality of their services. And even in those cases, people are likely to be included—for instance, by surveying or observing them.

Because people are almost always involved in evaluations, concerns arise over how their participation and the information they provide will be protected. Almost all nations subscribe to some form of guidance for human subjects' protection, as do school and health care systems and other for-profit and nonprofit institutions. Many journals will only publish evaluation reports if the evaluator provides evidence that human subjects' protection guidance was followed. The following discussion focuses on the United States; however, the principles are applicable and are used throughout the world.

Evaluations That Need Institutional Review or Ethics Board Approval

If you intend to conduct an evaluation for a public or private nonprofit or for-profit organization or institution that receives U.S. government support (even if you are a student), then you are likely to have to get approval from an institutional review board, or IRB, before you can begin. The IRB oversees reviewing the design of your evaluation study to guarantee that it is structured in a way that will protect each participant's privacy and other rights. If the IRB approves, you can proceed with the evaluation. If it does not, you will not be allowed to collect data. Although various state and local institutional review boards may differ in their specific requirements, nearly all major social, health, and welfare agencies within and outside of the U.S. have standards in place for the protection of human research subjects.

An IRB is an administrative body whose purpose is to protect the rights and welfare of individuals who are recruited to participate in research activities. According to the U.S. government, all IRB activities related to human subjects research should be guided by the ethical principles published in "The Belmont Report: Ethical Principles and Guidelines for the Protection of Human Subjects of Research" (www.hhs.gov/ohrp/regulations-and-policy/belmont-report). This report, which was prepared by the National Commission for the Protection of Human Subjects of Biomedical and Behavioral Research in 1979, is the foundation for ethical standards in all research involving human subjects, including evaluation. Three major principles come from "The Belmont Report":

- *Respect for persons.* This principle incorporates at least two ethical convictions: First, that individuals should be treated as autonomous agents; and second, that persons with diminished autonomy (e.g., very young children or people with dementing illnesses) are entitled to protection.
- *Beneficence.* This principle holds that researchers must treat research participants in an ethical manner, not only by respecting their decisions and protecting them from harm, but also by actively making efforts to secure their well-being.
- *Justice.* This principle concerns the balance for research participants between receiving the benefits of research and bearing its burdens. For example, to ensure justice, researchers need to examine their selection of research subjects to determine whether they are systematically choosing persons from some classes (e.g., welfare recipients, persons in institutions) simply because of those individuals' easy availability rather than for reasons directly related to the problems being studied.

U.S. government policy mandates that an IRB must have at least five members and that the members must have varied backgrounds. When selecting IRB members, an institution must consider the racial and cultural heritage of potential members and must be sensitive to community attitudes. In addition to possessing the professional competence necessary to review specific research activities, IRB members must be able to ascertain the acceptability of proposed research in terms of institutional commitments and regulations, applicable law, and standards of professional conduct and practice.

U.S. government policy also requires that if an IRB regularly reviews research that involves subjects within vulnerable categories (such as children, prisoners, pregnant women, or physically or mentally disabled persons), the institution must consider including among the IRB's members one or more individuals who are knowledgeable about and experienced in working with such subjects. Also, the institution must make every effort to ensure that its IRB consists of a mix of male and female members.

Evaluations That Are Exempt from Ethics Board Approval

A program evaluation is *research* (and thus needs IRB approval) when the evaluator intends to create generalizable knowledge that will be shared outside of the program being evaluated, whether in professional presentations, reports, or published articles. Process and implementation evaluations are less likely to require IRB approval than those focusing on effectiveness, quality, and value because the data gathered in those evaluations is typically used only to assess progress and to identify areas for improvement within programs. Example 1.12 describes an evaluation for which institutional review board (IRB) approval is not required.

Example 1.12 An Evaluation for Which IRB Approval Is Not Required

A community health center wants to improve its rate of vaccination to prevent influenza. A system is set up to remind physicians which of their patients is due for the vaccination. The health center conducts an evaluation of the effectiveness of the reminder system, collecting data each year for two years. Information from the evaluation is not shared outside the health center.

The evaluation in Example 1.12 is not considered to be research because the findings are used only by the health center. Evaluations of this type (which focus on the progress of a program—here, the reminder system) are called *quality improvement evaluations* because their purpose is to improve deficiencies in health care quality. In this case, the inadequacy is the poor rate of delivery of a vaccination that is recommended for most people by many national and international agencies.

What the IRB Will Review

When determining whether an evaluation can be implemented, an IRB will consider all the elements listed below.

If your evaluation is considered research, the IRB will ask to review the following documents:

- **Advance texts, emails, and letters:** Are you sending texts, emails, or letters to members of the community supporting the evaluation and recommending participation? If so, the IRB will need to review the contents.
- **Posters or flyers:** Are you planning to post notices inviting participation? Are you going to prepare flyers to post online or hand out at schools, clinics, or health fairs? If so, the IRB will need to review the contents.
- **Screening scripts:** Will you be screening potential participants to determine if they meet the criteria for inclusion in the evaluation? Will you be asking people to give their ages or

---

Criteria Used by the Institutional Review Board

✓ **Study design:** Many experts agree that the IRB should only approve studies that are valid and of value. Poorly designed studies necessarily produce biased results. Study design includes how subjects or participants are recruited, selected, and assigned to groups; the reliability and validity of measures or instruments; and the method of data analysis.

✓ **Risks and benefits:** The IRB evaluates whether the risks to participants are reasonable in relation to the anticipated benefits, if any, to the participants, as well as the importance of the knowledge reasonably expected to result from the evaluation.

✓ **Equitable selection of participants:** The IRB usually considers the purpose and setting of the evaluation and closely examines any proposed study involving vulnerable subject populations, such as children, prisoners, persons with cognitive disorders, or economically or educationally disadvantaged persons.

✓ **Identification of participants and confidentiality:** The IRB reviews the researcher's planned methods for prospective identification of participants, for identifying and contacting potential participants, and for ensuring participants' privacy and confidentiality.

✓ **Qualifications:** The IRB examines the qualifications of the evaluator and the evaluation team. In addition, the IRB considers the adequacy of the facilities and equipment to be used in conducting the research and maintaining the rights and welfare of the participants.

✓ **Informed consent:** The process of obtaining participants' informed consent to their participation in the evaluation goes to the heart of the matter of ethical research. The IRB often focuses a great deal of attention on the issue of informed consent.

describe their personal behaviors? Regardless of how you approach people (in person, by email, through social media, or on the phone), the IRB will need to review the details of your planned approach, including any scripts used for screening.

- **Informed consent forms:** Once you have determined that a potential participant is eligible, willing, and able to participate; you must give him or her opportunity to decide freely whether to participate. To do this, you must provide the potential subject with complete information about the research through an informed consent form. The IRB will need to review this form.

Informed Consent

Purpose

When participants give their *informed consent* to participate in a program evaluation, it means that they are knowledgeable about the risks and benefits of participation and the activities that participating entails. They also agree to the terms of participation and are knowledgeable about their rights as research participants.

Participants are often required to acknowledge their informed consent to participate in writing. If you cannot obtain a participant's signature on an informed consent form (e.g., if your only contact with the participant is over the phone), then you must be able to provide evidence that the contents of the form were explained to the participant, and that he or she understood them. Informed consent forms are designed to protect all parties: the subject, the evaluator, and the institution. Therefore, it is important that such forms present information in a well-organized and easily understood format.

If your evaluation includes children, you may have to design separate informed consent forms for their parents and assent (verbal) forms for the children. If your evaluation does not include children, the IRB may ask you to justify their exclusion.

Contents of an Informed Consent Form to Participate in an Evaluation

The required contents of informed consent forms vary from institution to institution, but the principles do not. Program evaluators should include all the elements shown in Example 1.13 in their informed consent forms.

Example 1.13 An Informed Consent Form for Participants in a Study of Alcohol Use and Health

Dear Participant,

The Foundation Clinic is taking part in an important research project conducted by university professors and sponsored by the National Institutes of Health. You have been asked to participate in this project because you told us over the phone that you are at least 65 years old, that you are planning to stay in the area and live in the community during the next 12 months, and that you have had at least one drink with alcohol in it during the past three months.

Your participation in the project is completely voluntary. If you decide not to participate, or if you agree and then change your mind before finishing, the care you receive at the Medical Foundation Clinic will not be affected in any way.

What is the project about?

Older adults become more sensitive to alcohol, and alcohol also interacts with medications used by older persons. The aim of the project is to see if educational reports can help you and your doctor understand more about alcohol use and its influence on health, medications, and physical and mental functioning among people 65 years of age and older.

What am I being asked to do?

The study has two parts. Today, you are being asked to participate in the first part of the study. For this part of the study, we would like you to complete a written questionnaire about your alcohol use, health, and use of health care. Please complete the questionnaire, sign this consent form, and mail both forms back to us in the accompanying prepaid envelope. The information you provide in this questionnaire will be analyzed for research purposes.

Some of the patients who participate in the first part of the study will be chosen for the second part of the study as well. If you are chosen for this next stage, we will be contacting you for more information over the next year.

At intervals three months, six months, and 12 months from now, we will ask you to complete questionnaires and mail them back to us. It will take you about 30–40 minutes to complete today's questionnaire, about 15–25 minutes to complete the second questionnaire, about 5–10 minutes to complete the third questionnaire, and about 25 to 30 minutes to complete the fourth questionnaire.

We also ask for your consent to give your personalized report of alcohol-related risks and problems to your doctor and to consult the administrative records to find out which medical services (if any) you used during the time being studied.

If you are asked and agree to participate in this second part of the study, you will be assigned to one of two groups of patients. The first group of patients will receive a booklet about alcohol use in older adults at the beginning of the study and will also receive periodic reports of their questionnaire results during the study. Patients assigned to the first group will be asked to read the reports and the booklet and will be called by a health educator to answer questions about the materials. The second group of patients will receive the same materials, but not until the end of the study.

Whether you are assigned to the first or the second group will depend on which group your doctor was randomly assigned to, and not on any decision made by the researchers or your physician.

Are there any risks or discomforts of participating in this project?

The only risks of participating in the project are the inconvenience of taking the time to answer the questions and review the report and the possibility that some of the questions on the questionnaire may worry or embarrass you. You are not required to answer any questions you may feel uncomfortable about answering. There are no medical procedures involved, and there is no financial cost to you associated with this study in any way, shape, or form.

What are the possible benefits?

The benefits of the study are the chance to learn about the possible risks of alcohol use and the possibility of improving the health education of other older adults. However, you might not benefit from participation in the study.

Will I be paid for my participation in the study?

To partially compensate you for your time, we will mail you $X in cash after you complete the first questionnaire. If you are chosen for the second part of the study, you will be paid $XX for the second questionnaire, $XY for the third questionnaire, and $YZ for the fourth questionnaire, for a total of $XYZ if you complete all the questionnaires.

How will my privacy be protected?

All the information you report is highly confidential and will be used only for study purposes. The consent form you sign will be filed in a locked storage cabinet during the project and shredded after completion of the project. Only the study's principal investigator, project manager, and the Medical Foundation Clinic data coordinators will have access to these files. All reports of information gained from your answers to the questionnaire will be shown as summaries of all participants' answers. No individual results will ever be used by the project team. All members of the team will be educated about the importance of protecting the privacy of patients and physicians.

Whom do I contact if I have any further questions?

You may call Dr. Lida Swan, the principal investigator, at 31X-794-ABCD, or email her at lswan@med.edu. Dr. Swan is Professor of Medicine and Public Health at the University of Eastwich. You may also contact Dr. Samuel Wygand, Professor of Medicine and Public Health, at 31X-459-DEFG, or Dr. John Tsai, Professor of Medicine, at 31X-459-UVWX. The project office is located in the Department of Medicine, Division of General Medicine and Evaluation, Box ABC, Eastwich, CA 90000.

What are my rights as a research subject?

You may withdraw your consent at any time and discontinue participation without penalty. You are not waiving any legal claims, rights, or remedies because of your participation in this research study. If you have questions regarding your rights as a research subject, contact the Office for Protection of Research Subjects, 832222 Humanities and Science Building, Box DEF, Eastwich, CA 90000; 31X-825-XYZA.

What if I agree to be in the study and then change my mind?

You can leave the project at any time. Again, the care you receive at the Medical Foundation Clinic will not be affected in any way if you decide to withdraw from the study.

How do I sign up?

If you want to join the project, please sign below on the line marked "Signature of Research Subject," write down the date next to your signature, and mail this form together with your completed questionnaire in the prepaid envelope provided. We will mail you a copy of the signed consent form.

Thank you very much for your interest in this research study!

SIGNATURE OF RESEARCH SUBJECT

Date of preparation:

IRB number:

Expiration date:

_____   _____
Signature of Research Subject   Date

SIGNATURE OF INVESTIGATOR

_____   _____
Signature of Investigator   Date

Notice that the participant is given a copy of the consent form. In mail and online surveys, a completed and returned questionnaire may be considered evidence of informed consent, but this depends on the rules laid down by the IRB and the purpose of the survey.

The Internet and Ethical Evaluations

Online data collection involves a web of computers that interact with one another. Communications take place between the evaluator and the participant, the participant and the web server, and the web server and the evaluator. Security breaches are possible anywhere within the web unless you put protections in place.

Communication between the Evaluator and the Participant

It is not uncommon for an evaluator to contact participants by email, text, or social media. The message will discuss the evaluation and invite the participant to click on a URL or paste it into their preferred browser. Unfortunately, email and other contact forms are not always secure or private. Many people are unaware of whether their computers or phones are secure or even how to secure them. Email programs maintained by employers often are not private. If people do not log off or are careless about passwords, their privacy can be compromised easily. Also, inadequate passwords are easy to crack. If you require people to use a password or passkey, you must ensure that the password set-up is secure. Social media have their own privacy guidelines, but as is well known, they are sometimes difficult to interpret and change.

Communication between the Participant and the Website

When a participant enters sensitive data in the blank spaces of a commonly used data collection measure like a web-based questionnaire, it is like a shopper providing a credit card number when shopping online. Reputable online merchants use a Secure Socket Layer (SSL) protocol that allows secure communications across the internet. An SSL protocol "encrypts" (converts into code) the user's input, and it "decrypts" it when it arrives at the website. Many potential participants are becoming aware of how easily their online responses can be intercepted unless they are secured, and without guarantees that responses are encrypted, some of them may refuse to participate. You must decide in advance whether to use SSL and how to explain your security choices to participants.

Communication between the Website and the Evaluator

Sensitive identifiable data needs to be protected in transit by using either an SSL protocol or a secure file transfer protocol.

Data Protection

Some people are reluctant to complete online data collection measures or even connect to them for fear that their privacy will be compromised. All databases storing sensitive and identifiable information must be protected, regardless of whether they are created and maintained by commercial firms or by individuals. Encrypting the databases probably provides the most security.

All reputable organizations develop or adapt rules for reassuring participants that privacy will be respected. Here are minimum criteria for a privacy policy for internet-based data collection:

If relevant, explain how cookies are used. Cookies are small amounts of information your browser stores. Cookies allow web-based applications to store information about selected items, user preferences, registration information, and other information that can be retrieved later. Are the cookies session-specific? If not, can users opt out of the web page feature that stores the cookies beyond the session?

Minimum Criteria for a Privacy Policy Using the Internet

Describe exactly which evaluation data will be stored in the evaluation's database.
Explain why any data is being stored.
Explain whether the organization gives, sells, or transfers information, and if it does, to whom and under which circumstances.
Tell how the site monitors unauthorized attempts to change the site's contents.
Discuss who maintains the site.

If you plan to use the internet to (1) communicate with study participants or (2) to send participant information to a collaborator or contractor, you should answer be able to complete this questionnaire for maintaining ethically sound online evaluation data collection.

Sample Questionnaire: Maintaining Ethically Sound Online Data Collection

1. Describe the measures that will be taken to ensure the Web server hosting the internet site is protected. In the description, provide information on physical security, firewalls, software patches/updates, and penetration drills.
2. If a password or other secure authorization method is to be used to allow access to the web site:
   - How will user passwords be distributed?
   - How will passwords and web access be terminated?
3. If the user session is encrypted, describe the method of encryption that will be used.
4. Explain who will have administrative access to data on the Web server. Give names, study roles, and organizational affiliations.
5. Explain in detail the administrative safeguards put in place to restrict unauthorized and unnecessary access.
6. Describe how the information will be used. Will you give, sell, or transfer information to anyone?
7. Give the name and address of the application owner—that is, the people who maintain the application.
8. If email is used to contact participants, describe the measures taken to assure participants that the communication is from an authorized person.
9. If participants are asked to contact the evaluators using email, describe how the participants will be authenticated to adequately ensure the source of the email communication.
10. Explain how the study consent form describes the potential risks to privacy associated with the use of email.
11. If email is to be used to send study data to investigators, vendors, or others, explain if and how the email will be encrypted.
12. If participants are to send you attachments by email, tell if they will be encrypted or password protected.
13. If automated email routing systems are used, describe the security controls that will be in place. Specifically, describe the testing and disaster recovery procedures.
14. If contractors or vendors have access to survey participants' personal identifiable or confidential information:
    - Describe the language that is included in the contract to protect participant privacy.
    - Describe the security requirements that will be provided to contractors or vendors who are designing or hosting web-based services for the evaluation.
15. Tell who on the evaluation team is responsible for ensuring that the outside organization's policies and procedures for confidentiality and security are followed. Provide the name of the person responsible and his/her professional position and affiliation.
16. Tell who is responsible for the general security administration for the information technology associated with each online data collection measure. Provide the name of the people responsible and their professional position and affiliation.

Each evaluation has different limits on what it needs to collect and from whom. Some evaluation participants are more vulnerable than others and need different safeguards.

Example 1.14 is an informed consent form typical of one that can be used in an online survey of teachers in a large school district. The survey's purpose is to identify needs for a program to improve morale in the school workplace.

Example 1.14 Consent Form for an Online Survey

Your individual responses to survey questions will be kept confidential by The Survey Project and its survey contractor, Online Systems, Inc. Confidential data is data that may not be released outside of The Survey Project with individual or school identification, except with permission from the participant. Individuals may grant The Survey Project permission to release confidential data that describes themselves. An authorized representative of a Survey Project member school may grant The Survey Project permission to release confidential data that describes his or her school. *[Comment: Defines and describes limits of confidentiality.]*

Online Systems, Inc. will generate aggregate reports that contain school-wide and departmental information to help your school identify, prioritize, and implement improvements in the school workplace that will increase student engagement. Information will not be reported in instances where participant groups contain fewer than five individuals. *[Comment: It may be possible to identify individual views in very small groups. This would violate privacy.]*

Data from open-ended questions will be provided to your school in de-identified, redacted form. Only de-identified record level data will be retained by The Survey Project, and only de-identified aggregate analyses will be shared in publications and research presentations with the academic community. *[Comment: How the data will be used.]* The Survey Project may release de-identified responses to individuals who agree to protect the data and who agree to The Survey Project's confidentiality policies. Online Systems, Inc. will store data on secure servers and will destroy all identified data within two years of survey administration. By participating, you will be contributing valuable information to your school. *[Comment: Servers will be secured. The vendor must destroy identifiable data within two years.]*

The Survey Project and Online Systems, Inc. have taken numerous steps to protect participants in The Survey Project. Ethics Board requirements require that you are informed that if the information collected were to become public with individual identification it could prove personally uncomfortable. *[Comment: This is a risk of participation.]*

This survey has been reviewed and approved according to The Survey Project's policies and procedures. By continuing, you acknowledge that you have read and understood the above information and agree to participate in this survey. *[Comment: This is an online survey, and the participant is not asked to "sign" to indicate willingness to participate. Signing software is available, but most evaluators will accept a completed survey as confirmation of informed consent.]* If you have any questions about the survey, contact… If you have any questions about your rights as a research participant, contact… *[Comment: Whom to contact with questions.]*

RESEARCH MISCONDUCT

Research misconduct is becoming an increasingly important concern throughout the world. Faking the data is a clear example of research misconduct. Subtler examples include the following:

- Exaggerating an evaluation's findings to support the evaluator's, funding agency's, or community's point of view.
- Changing the evaluation protocol or method of implementation without informing the IRB or ethics board before doing so.

Table 1.1 Problematic Research Behaviors

Problematic Behavior	Definition
Misconduct	Fabrication, falsification, or plagiarism.
Questionable research practices	Actions that violate values of research that may be detrimental to the research process, but which do not directly threaten the integrity of the research record.
	Examples include failing to retain research records for a reasonable period and using inappropriate statistics to enhance findings.
Other misconduct, not pertaining to scientific integrity	Unacceptable behaviors that are subject to generally applicable legal and social penalties, but which are not unique to research.
	Examples include sexual harassment, misuse of funds, and violations of local or national regulations.
Other misconduct, pertaining to scientific integrity	Unacceptable behavior that does not directly affect the integrity of the research process but is nevertheless directly associated with misconduct in science.
	Examples include cover-ups of scientific misconduct and reprisals against whistleblowers.
Sloppiness	Negligent or irregular research practices that risk distortion of the research record but lack the intent to do so.
	Examples include failure to keep adequate project records and maintain an accessible database with a complete operations manual.

- Failing to maintain adequate documentation of the evaluation's methods (e.g., by neglecting to prepare a codebook or operations manual).
- Releasing participant information without permission to do so.
- Having insufficient resources to complete the evaluation as promised.
- Having financial or other interests in common with the funding agencies or supporters of the evaluation (conflict of interest).

Table 1.1 lists and defines some of the problematic research behaviors that may occur in many situations in which evaluations are conducted.

MANAGING EVALUATION RESOURCES

Program Evaluation Job Description

Evaluators work for academic institutions, government agencies, private industry, and nonprofit organizations. As businesses become more data-driven, the need for program evaluators who can gather and analyze data is likely to increase because data-driven decision-making is becoming increasingly important in all industries. Evaluators may work in an office although they may also travel to the worksites of the programs they are evaluating, and these worksites may be in another city or country.

Program evaluations are typically performed by interdisciplinary teams because of the diverse skills needed to do an excellent job. For instance, it is not unusual for an evaluation to need talented people who can do sophisticated psychometrics while also needing others who can create graphically engaging and accurate reports of statistical findings.

A job description for a program evaluator will ask for people with knowledge of and expertise in the following:

1. Program evaluation principles such as identifying and justifying evidence of effectiveness, quality, and value. This can mean having the ability to conduct focus groups and organize professional and community conferences to assist in the evidence-setting process. The evaluator should also have skills in doing systematic literature reviews and meta-analyses to justify the evidence used to support program findings and the methods used to collect and analyze data.
2. Designing studies to include the selection and implementation of research designs and sampling strategies that minimize bias.
3. Designing ethical studies that respect each participant and protect their privacy and well-being.
4. Collecting, managing, and analyzing data including identifying valid measures (psychometrics), organizing the evaluation's databases, and conducting statistical and qualitative analysis.
5. Communicating evaluation methods and findings in person and in writing to stakeholders within and outside the evaluation setting.
6. Working productively with stakeholders including funding agencies, policymakers, researchers, and the community.
7. Managing the evaluation including hiring, training, and supervising staff.
8. Working independently and as part of a team.
9. Understanding the program's substantive content (such as the learning, business, or health behavior models that are its instructional foundations).
10. Creating and following a budget that supports the evaluation team.

Some job descriptions may have additional requirements such as requiring evaluators to be able to speak another language and be willing to travel to other countries for extended periods of time.

Program Evaluation Budgets (and Timelines)

The format for describing and justifying an evaluation's budget will differ across countries and even sites. Also, some evaluators are responsible for putting the entire evaluation budget together, while others have only a minimal role, if any, in preparing it. And not all funding agencies use the same budgeting categories. It is important, however, that all evaluation personnel have knowledge of what the total budget is and what it includes. The following is a checklist to consider when preparing or reviewing an evaluation's budget.

✓ **Learn about direct costs.**
These include all salaries and benefits, supplies, travel, and equipment.
✓ **Decide on the number of days (or hours) that constitute a working year.**
Commonly used numbers in the U.S. are 230 days (1,840 hours) and 260 days (2,080 hours) for a working year. You use these numbers to show the proportion of time, or "level of effort," given by each staff member. Example: People who spend 20% of their time on the evaluation (assuming 260 days per year) are spending 0.20 x 260—that is, 52 days, or 416 hours.
✓ **Create a timeline in terms of months to complete each evaluation task (Example 1.15).**
Example: Software development will take place from August 2024 through February 2025.
Example: Patient surveys will occur in April 2025 and also in August 2027.

Example 1.15 Portions of a Timeline for a Four-Year Program Evaluation

Year 1	8 24	9 24	10 24	11 24	12 24	1 25	2 25	3 25	4 25	5 25	6 25	7 25
Study set-up (e.g., recruitment materials; site preparation)	X	X	X	X	X	X	X					
Software development	X	X	X	X	X	X	X					
Data management system preparation	X	X	X	X	X	X	X					
Baseline provider survey							X					
Provider training							X					
Subject recruitment								X	X	X	X	X
Program Implementation								X	X	X	X	X
Patient surveys								X	X	X	X	X
Quality assurance (training, implementation, monitoring)								X	X	X	X	X
Data management, cleaning and programming								X	X	X	X	X
Year 4	**8 27**	**9 27**	**10 27**	**11 27**	**12 27**	**1 28**	**2 28**	**3 28**	**4 28**	**5 28**	**6 28**	**7 28**
Patient surveys	X	X	X	X	X	X	X					
Quality assurance (training, implementation, monitoring)	X	X	X	X	X	X	X					
Data management, cleaning, and programming	X	X	X	X	X	X	X	X				

✓ **Estimate the number of days (or hours) you need each person to complete each task.**
Example: Jones, 10 days; Smith, 8 days. If required, convert the days into hours and compute an hourly rate (e.g., Jones: 10 days, or 80 hours).

✓ **Compute a person's daily (and hourly) rate.**
Example: Jones, US $/EUR per day, or US $/EUR per hour; Smith, US $/EUR per day, or US $/EUR per hour.

✓ **Remember to include costs of "benefits" (e.g., vacation, pension, and health)—usually a percentage of the salary.**
Example: Benefits are 25% of Jones's salary. For example, the cost of benefits for ten days of Jones's time is 10 x US $or 10 x EUR per day x 0.25.

✓ **Carefully plan to include the costs of other expenses that are incurred specifically for this evaluation.**
Example: One two-hour focus group with ten participants costs US $/EUR. Each participant gets a US $/EUR honorarium for a total of US $/EUR; refreshments cost US $/EUR;

a focus group expert facilitator costs US $/EUR; the materials costs US $/EUR for reproduction, notebooks, nametags.

✓ **Do not forget the indirect costs, or the costs that are incurred to keep the study team going.**
Every individual and institution has indirect costs. Indirect costs are often a prescribed percentage of the total cost of the evaluation (e.g., 10%). Example: All routine costs of doing "business," such as workers' compensation and other insurance; attorney's and license fees; utilities, rent, and supplies; and hardware and software maintenance.

✓ **If the evaluation lasts more than one year, build in cost-of-living increases. Be prepared to justify all costs in writing.**
Document all costs relevant to the evaluation. This includes license fees for survey software, office supplies, and postage costs.

SUMMARY AND TRANSITION TO THE NEXT CHAPTER ON EVALUATION QUESTIONS AND EVIDENCE OF PROGRAM EFFECTIVENESS, QUALITY, AND VALUE

Program evaluation aims to be an unbiased, scientifically based investigation into a program's effectiveness, quality, and value. An unbiased evaluation is free from systematic errors which are the result of misdirected purpose and flawed study designs and data analysis. An effective program provides measurable benefits to individuals, communities, and societies, and these benefits are greater than their human and financial costs. A high-quality program evaluation meets its users' needs and is based on sound theory and the best available research evidence. A program's value is measured by its worth to individuals, the community, and society.

Evaluators are responsible for posing justifiable evaluation questions and deciding and justifying evidence of effectiveness, quality, and value; choosing unbiased study designs and sampling methods; and collecting, analyzing, interpreting, and reporting information. The information produced by program evaluations is used by the financial supporters of the programs as well as by consumers (patients, students, teachers, and health care professionals), program developers, policy makers, and other evaluators.

Collecting and analyzing interim or formative evaluation data is expensive and may produce misleading results; evaluators who choose to collect interim data should proceed with caution. However, formative evaluation data is helpful in determining the feasibility and its associated evaluation methodology. Process or implementation evaluations are useful because they provide data on what and when program activities occurred, factors that clarify the program's dynamics.

Evaluations may use qualitative or statistical data or both in the same study. Participatory evaluations involve stakeholders in all phases of the evaluation. Comparative effectiveness evaluations compare two existing programs in naturalistic settings and provide information to help evaluation stakeholders make informed choices about which one to choose.

Evaluators must follow internationally accepted ethics principles by respecting the uniqueness and independence of individuals, securing their well-being, and balancing the risks and benefits of participation in evaluation studies. Part of conducting ethical evaluations is to recognize research misconduct which includes plagiarism and sloppiness in adhering to rigorous research practices.

Evaluators have a complex job. A typical job description for hiring a program evaluator includes skills in conducting evaluation projects, communicating with stakeholders, implementing valid research designs and measurement strategies, and supervising project management. Evaluators are also responsible for following a budget and a timeline for accomplishing all evaluation tasks.

Before evaluators can decide on the evaluation's design and data collection methods, they must choose and justify evaluation questions and decide on what constitutes evidence of program effectiveness, quality, and value. The next chapter discusses how to select and state evaluation questions and choose appropriate, justifiable evidence.

EXERCISES: CHAPTER 1

Exercise 1

Directions

Define program evaluation.

Exercise 2

Directions

Read the two evaluation summaries below and, using only the information offered, answer these questions:

1. What are the evaluation questions?
2. What is the evidence of effectiveness, quality, or value?
3. What data collection measures are being used?

Evaluation 1: The "Families First" Program to Prevent Child Abuse: Results of a Cluster Randomized Controlled Trial in West Java, Indonesia (Ruiz-Casares et al., 2022)

Objective: To evaluate the" Families First" program in West Java, Indonesia.
Program: The "Families First" parenting program is a ten-week paraprofessional-administered adaptation of the Positive Discipline in Everyday Parenting program for West Java, Indonesia. The evaluators randomly assigned 20 rural and urban villages in West Java, Indonesia, to be part of the program or to stay on a waitlist. The primary outcome was presence versus absence of caregiver-reported physical or emotional punishment immediately post-intervention. Between 2017 and 2018, measurements were taken before randomization, immediately post-intervention, and six months post-intervention. A total of 374 caregivers in the ten intervention villages and 362 in the ten waitlist villages were included in the trial and in outcome analyses.
Results: Being in the program did not result in a lower proportion of intervention families using punishment immediately post-intervention. There were no significant differences for "positive and involved parenting, setting limits, and opinion on discipline," but caregivers in the intervention group had significantly lower odds of using "positive discipline." The evaluators concluded that "Families First" did not prevent punishment in a setting with low levels of reported punishment but suggested that the program should be tested in a setting with higher levels or among at-risk people.

Evaluation 2: Evaluating a Mental Health Intervention for Schoolchildren Exposed to Violence: A Randomized Controlled Trial (Stein et al., 2003)

Objective: To evaluate the effectiveness of a collaboratively designed school-based intervention for reducing children's symptoms of posttraumatic stress disorder (PTSD) and depression that resulted from exposure to violence.
Program: Students were randomly assigned to a ten-session standardized cognitive-behavioral therapy (the Cognitive-Behavioral Intervention for Trauma in Schools) early intervention group or to a waitlist delayed intervention comparison group conducted by trained school mental health clinicians.
Results: The evaluators found that compared with the waitlist delayed intervention group (no intervention), after three months of intervention, students who were randomly assigned to the

early intervention group had significantly lower scores on the Child PTSD Symptom Scale, the Child Depression Inventory, Pediatric Symptom Checklist, and the Teacher-Child Rating Scale. Six months after both groups had received the intervention, the differences between the two groups were not significantly different for symptoms of PTSD and depression.

Exercise 3

Directions

Explain whether each of these is an evaluation study or not.

a. The purpose of the study was to evaluate a randomized culturally tailored program to prevent high-HIV-risk sexual behaviors for women residing in urban areas.
b. The researchers aimed to determine the effectiveness of a program to prevent the use of tobacco. The program was specifically designed to promote tobacco cessation and discourage starting smoking among male secondary school athletes.
c. To study drivers' exposure to distractions, unobtrusive video camera units were installed in the vehicles of 70 volunteer drivers over six one-week time periods.

Exercise 4

Directions

The following is an informed consent form for a hypothetical diabetes self-care program. Parts of the form are completed, but others are not. Using the descriptions provided, complete the form by writing in the needed content.

Informed Consent Form for the Diabetes Self-Care Program

You are asked to take part in three telephone interviews and three self-administered questionnaires on your general health, your quality of life since being diagnosed with diabetes, and the quality of health care you have received while in the program. Robert Fung, MD, MPH, is directing the project. Dr. Fung works in the Department of Medicine at the University of East Hampton. You are being asked to take part in the interviews and questionnaires because you are enrolled in the Diabetes Self-Care Program.

1. Tell eligible subjects that participation is voluntary, they can leave whenever they choose, and their health care will not be affected.

Disclosure Statement

Your health care provider may be an investigator in this study protocol. As an investigator, he/she is interested in both your clinical welfare and your responses to the interview questions. Before entering this study or at any time during the study, you may ask for a second opinion about your care from another doctor who is in no way associated with the Diabetes Self-Care Program. You are not under any obligation to take part in any research project offered by your physician.

Reason for the Telephone Interviews and Self-Administered Questionnaires

The interviews and the questionnaires are being done for the following reason: to find out if the Diabetes Self-Care Program is meeting the needs of the patients enrolled in the program.

During the telephone interview, a trained member of the Diabetes Self-Care Program staff will ask you a series of questions about your health, your quality of life since being diagnosed with diabetes, and the quality of the health care you have received while in the Diabetes Self-Care Program.

The self-administered survey questions will cover the same topics, but you will be able to answer them on your own and in any place that is convenient for you.

2. Tell participants that the program will use their answers (and answers from others) to find out about the appropriateness of services and any needed changes.

What You Will Be Asked to Do

If you agree to take part in this study, you will be asked to do the following things:

1. Answer three short (20-minute) telephone interviews. The telephone interviewer will ask you general questions about your health, your quality of life since you were diagnosed with diabetes, and the quality of health care you have received while in the Diabetes Self-Care Program. You will be called to complete an interview when you first enroll in the program, six months after your enrollment, and when you leave the program. The interviews will be completed at whatever time is best for you.

Sample Questions

How confident are you in your ability to know what questions to ask a doctor?
    During the PAST FOUR WEEKS, how much did diabetes interfere with your normal work (including both work outside the home and housework)?
    Would you say not at all, a little bit, moderately, quite a bit, or extremely?

2. Answer three short (20-minute) self-administered questionnaires. The self-administered questionnaires will ask you general questions about your health, your quality of life since you were diagnosed with diabetes, and the quality of health care you have received while in the Diabetes Self-Care Program. The self-administered questionnaires will be mailed to you when you first enroll in the program, six months after your enrollment, and when you leave the program. You can complete the self-administered questionnaires at whatever times are best for you. You will be provided with a prepaid envelope in which to return each questionnaire.

Sample Questions

How many drinks of alcohol did you usually drink each day during the past four weeks? (None, one, two, three, or four or more)
    On a scale of 1 (very confident) to 6 (not at all confident), how confident are you in your ability to know what questions to ask a doctor?

3. If you do not understand a question or have a problem with a self-administered questionnaire, you will be asked to call Ms. Estella Ruiz at the Diabetes Self-Care Program office at 1-800-000-0000. She will be able to assist you.

Possible Risks and Discomforts

3. Tell respondents that the surveys may include questions about their physical or emotional health or their experience with the program that they may feel sensitive about answering, and that they do not have to answer questions that bother them.

Potential Benefits to Subjects and/or to Society

The purpose of the telephone interviews and self-administered questionnaires is to improve the services that the Diabetes Self-Care Program provides to the patients enrolled in the program.

Your responses might lead to changes in the program that would improve the services that the Diabetes Self-Care Program provides.

Payment for Taking Part

4. Tell participants that they will not be paid for their time.

Confidentiality

Any information that is collected from you and that can be identified with you will remain confidential. Your identity will not be revealed to anyone outside the research team unless we have your permission or as required by law. You will not be identified in any reports or presentations. Confidentiality will be maintained in the following ways:

1. All your interviews and questionnaires will be coded with a number that identifies you. Your name will not be on any of these materials.
2. A master list of names and code numbers will be kept in a separate, confidential, password-protected computer database.
3. All copies of the self-administered questionnaires will be kept in a locked file cabinet in a locked research office.
4. All telephone interviews will be recorded in a confidential computer database.
5. When analysis of the data is conducted, your name will not be associated with your data in any way.
6. Only research staff will have access to these files.

Taking Part and Choosing Not to Take Part in Telephone Interviews and Self-Administered Questionnaires

5. Tell participants that it is up to them whether they want to take part and that, if they do, they can stop at any time and their health care will not be affected.

Identification of Investigators

If you have concerns or questions about this study, please contact Robert Funk, MD, MPH, by mailing inquiries to Box 000, Los Angeles, CA 90000-9990. Dr. Funk can also be reached by telephone at 1-800-000-0000 or by email at rfunk@medmail.edu.

Rights of Participants

You may choose to end your agreement to take part in the telephone interviews and self-administered questionnaires at any time. You may stop taking part without penalty. You are not giving up any legal claims, rights, or remedies because you take part in the telephone interviews and self-administered questionnaires. If you have questions about your rights as a research subject, contact the Office for Protection of Research Subjects, 2107 QQQ Building, Box 951694, East Hampton, CA 90273, 1-800-123-XYZZ.

I understand the events described above. My questions have been answered to my satisfaction, and I agree to take part in this study. I have been given a copy of this form.

Name of Subject (Please Print)

_____   _____

Signature of Subject   Date

REFERENCES AND SUGGESTED READINGS

Codjia, P., Kutondo, E., Kamudoni, P., et al. (2022). Mid-term evaluation of Maternal and Child Nutrition Programme (MCNP II) in Kenya. *BMC Public Health, 22*(1): 2191.

Coulton, S., Stockdale, K., Marchand, C., et al. (2017). Pragmatic randomised controlled trial to evaluate the effectiveness and cost effectiveness of a multi-component intervention to reduce substance use and risk-taking behaviour in adolescents involved in the criminal justice system: A trial protocol (RISKIT-CJS). *BMC Public Health, 17*(1): 246.

Galvagno, S.M., Jr., Haut, E.R., Zafar, S.N., et al. (2012). Association between helicopter vs ground emergency medical services and survival for adults with major trauma. *JAMA: The Journal of the American Medical Association, 307*(*15*): 1602–1610.

Gillam, S.L, Vaughn, S., Roberts, G., et al. (2023). Improving oral and written narration and reading comprehension of children at-risk for language and literacy difficulties: Results of a randomized clinical trial. *Journal of Educational Psychology, 115*: 99–117.

Hardy, L.L., King, L., Kelly, B., Farrell, L., & Howlett, S. (2010). Munch and Move: Evaluation of a preschool healthy eating and movement skill program. *The International Journal of Behavioral Nutrition and Physical Activity, 7*: 80.

Le Roux, K.W., Almirol, E., Rezvan, P.H., et al. (2020). Community health workers impact on maternal and child health outcomes in rural South Africa—a non-randomized two-group comparison study. *BMC Public Health, 20*(1): 1404.

Lundström, L., Flygare, O., Andersson, E., et al. (2022). Effect of internet-based vs face-to-face cognitive behavioral therapy for adults with obsessive-compulsive disorder: A randomized clinical trial. *JAMA Network Open, 5*(3): e221967–e221967.

Marczinski, C.A. & Stamates. A.L. (2013). Artificial sweeteners versus regular mixers increase breath alcohol concentrations in male and female social drinkers. *Alcoholism, Clinical and Experimental Research, 37*(4): 696–702.

Stein, B.D., Jaycox, L.H., Kataoka, S.H., Wong, M., Tu, W., Elliott, M.N., & Fink, A. (2003). A mental health intervention for schoolchildren exposed to violence: A randomized controlled trial. *JAMA: The Journal of the American Medical Association, 290*(5): 603–611.

Ruiz-Casares, M., Thombs, B.D., Mayo, N.E., Andrina, M., Scott, S.C., & Platt, R.W. (2022). The Families First Program to prevent child abuse: Results of cluster randomized controlled trial in West Java, Indonesia. *Prevention Science, 23*(8): 1457–1469.

Volpp, K.G., Loewenstein, G., & Asch, D.A. (2012). Assessing value in health care programs. *JAMA: The Journal of the American Medical Association, 307*(20): 2153–2154.

Yu, S. (2012). College students' justification for digital piracy: A mixed methods study. *Journal of Mixed Methods Research, 6*(4): 364–378.

Suggested Websites

Instruction for Conducting Program Evaluations
www.cdc.gov/evaluation/index.htm

The U.S. Centers for Disease Control Evaluation Model
www.youtube.com/watch?v=tOjieBh1ce0

How to Do a Cost Analysis
www.wikihow.com/Do-a-Cost-Analysis

Comprehensive List of Databases to look for publications on evaluation topics
https://en.wikipedia.org/wiki/List_of_academic_databases_and_search_engines

Discussion of Bias
www.ncbi.nlm.nih.gov/pmc/articles/PMC2917255
https://training.cochrane.org/handbook/current

Stakeholder Engagement
www.betterevaluation.org/frameworks-guides/rainbow-framework/manage/understand-engage-stakeholders

CDC's Evaluation Framework Step One: Engaging Stakeholders
https://campusmentalhealth.ca/toolkits/evaluation/planning/building-an-evaluation-plan/engage-stakeholders
https://campusmentalhealth.ca/toolkits/evaluation/planning/building-an-evaluation-plan/engage-stakeholders

For Ethical Evaluations
www.apa.org/research/responsible/human
www.hhs.gov/ohrp/regulations-and-policy/regulations/common-rule/index.html

World Health Organization
www.who.int/activities/ensuring-ethical-standards-and-procedures-for-research-with-human-beings
www.wma.net/what-we-do/medical-ethics/declaration-of-helsinki
www.eval.org/About/Guiding-Principles
https://europeanevaluation.org

To Learn More about Evaluation Research, Practice and Career Opportunities
American Evaluation Association—www.eval.org
Canadian Evaluation Society—https://evaluationcanada.ca
European Evaluation Society—https://europeanevaluation.org

ANSWERS TO THE EXERCISES: CHAPTER 1

Exercise 1

An evaluation is a systematic assessment of a program's *effectiveness*, *quality*, and *value*. High-quality evaluations are scientific studies that result in unbiased evidence of the program's achievements, impact, and costs. Stakeholders use evaluation information to better understand their program and to make informed decisions about program improvement, continuation, and funding.

An effective program achieves positive outcomes and provides measurable benefits to its target population. In an effective program, the benefits are greater than their human and financial costs. A high-quality program meets its stakeholders' needs and is based on sound theory and the best available research evidence. A program's value is measured by its costs and its worth to its stakeholders and society. Each program evaluation must decide whether it will investigate effectiveness, quality, or value—or all three, a decision sometimes made jointly with stakeholders.

Exercise 2

1. Evaluating the Effectiveness of the "Families First" Program

Evaluation Question
Does a difference exist in reported physical or emotional punishment between caregivers before and after participation in the adapted Positive Discipline in Everyday Parenting Program when compared to a random selection of waitlist controls?

Evidence
1. Participating parents will use punishment significantly less than non-participating families after completing the program ("post-intervention").
2. Participating families will provide significantly greater evidence of "positive and involved parenting, setting limits, and opinion on discipline."

Data Collection Measures
Caregiver-reported physical or emotional punishment. Reports are given immediately before and after program participation and six months later.

2. Evaluating a Mental Health Intervention for Schoolchildren Exposed to Violence: A Randomized Controlled Trial

Evaluation Question
Did the program achieve its objectives of reducing PTSD, depression, symptoms, and teacher-perceived behavior?

Evidence
At a six-month follow-up, after both groups receive the intervention, no difference is found between experimental and control groups.

Data Collection Methods
The Child PTSD Symptom Scale, the Child Depression Inventory, Pediatric Symptom Checklist, and the Teacher-Child Rating Scale

Exercise 3

a. Yes. This is an evaluation study. The program is an intervention to prevent high-HIV-risk sexual behaviors for women in urban areas.
b. Yes. This is an evaluation study. The intervention is a spit tobacco intervention.
c. No. This is not an evaluation study. The researchers are not analyzing the effectiveness, quality, or value of a program or intervention.

Exercise 4

Informed consent for the diabetes self-care program

Tell eligible participants that participation is voluntary, they can leave whenever they choose, and their health care will not be affected.

Reason for the telephone interviews and self-administered questionnaires

Tell participants that the program will use their answers (and answers from others) to find out about the appropriateness of services and needed changes.

Possible risks and discomforts

Tell participants that the surveys may include questions about their physical or emotional health or their experience with the program which they may feel sensitive about answering. Tell them that they do not have to answer questions that bother them.

Payment for taking part

Tell participants that they will not be paid for their time.

*Taking part and choosing not to take part in telephone interviews
and self-administered questionnaires*

Tell participants that it is up to them whether they take part and that, if they do, they can stop at any time, and their health care will not be affected.

CHAPTER 2 | EVALUATION QUESTIONS AND EVIDENCE OF EFFECTIVENESS, QUALITY, AND VALUE

PURPOSE OF CHAPTER 2

A program evaluation aims to be an unbiased investigation of a program's effectiveness, quality, and value. Evaluations answer questions like: Did the program benefit all participants? Did the benefits endure? Is the program sustainable? Did the program meet the needs of the community, and was it done more efficiently than current practice?

Evaluations can answer many questions, and the evaluator must compile a list that is comprehensive enough to be meaningful and answerable on time and within budget. Moreover, the answers to program evaluation questions require not just a "yes" or a "no," but evidence for the answers. Unbiased evidence is the result of rigorous research designs, valid data collection, and appropriate data analysis methods that are specifically linked to the evaluation questions.

This chapter begins with a discussion of commonly asked evaluation questions and their associated hypotheses. Evaluation questions focus on programs, participants, outcomes, impact, and costs and provide data on whether a program achieves its objectives, in what context, with whom, and at what cost. The answers to the questions provide evidence for a program's effectiveness, quality, and value. The questions must therefore be comprehensive and cover all aspects of the program that are important to the evaluation's users and funders.

Evidence of program effectiveness, quality, and value is often based on statistical significance. For example, a program is considered effective if the participants in the new program benefit more than participants in an older program, and the effects are not likely due to chance as determined by statistical tests of significance. But, for the evidence to be useful, it should also have practical or clinical meaning. That is, the effect should be large enough so that it is important to everyone who has an interest in the evaluation's findings. Sources of practical or clinical importance include experts, stakeholders, and the research literature.

The relationships among the evaluation questions and hypotheses, evaluation evidence, and independent and dependent variables are also examined in this chapter. Their connection is illustrated using a special reporting form: The QEV or Questions, Evidence, Variables Report.

A READER'S GUIDE TO CHAPTER 2

Evaluation Questions and Hypotheses
    Evaluation Questions
    Evaluation Hypotheses
    Evaluation Questions: Program Goals and Objectives
    Evaluation Questions: Participants

DOI: 10.4324/9781032635071-2

EVALUATION QUESTIONS AND HYPOTHESES

Evaluation Questions

Evaluations can answer many questions about a program, but regardless of which ones are selected or how many of them there are, their combined answers must provide a comprehensive assessment of effectiveness, quality, or merit. An effectiveness evaluation that asks if a program achieved beneficial outcomes with all its participants may not be sufficiently comprehensive if it neglects to ask if the benefits endure over time.

An evaluation can provide information about a program's political and economic environment and accomplishments, the participants' personal characteristics and behaviors, and the financial and human costs and benefits of program implementation. The challenge for the evaluation team is to identify evaluation questions whose answers will provide comprehensive and useful information and to be able to do so within the available time and money. To identify a comprehensive list of evaluation questions, evaluators usually rely on the literature and consultation with subject matter experts, other evaluators, and stakeholders including the community, program developers, and funding agencies.

Being able to justify the choice of evaluation questions and provide evidence of how they were selected is indicative of a rigorous evaluation. Justification is especially important if the evaluation's findings are negative, or the program is contentious.

Evaluation Hypotheses

Evaluation questions are often accompanied by hypotheses. A question that asks if a program achieves equal benefits for all participants at the same cost may be accompanied by hypotheses such as: "No difference in program benefits or costs will be found between men and women," or "Younger people will benefit more than older people but at increased cost."

Almost all evaluations directly or indirectly ask the question: Did the program achieve its goals and objectives?

Evaluation Questions: Program Goals and Objectives

A program's goals are usually relatively general and long-term, as shown in Example 2.1.

Example 2.1 Typical Program Goals

For the public or the community at large:

- Optimize health status, education, and well-being.
- Improve quality of life.
- Foster improved physical, social, and psychological functioning.
- Support new knowledge about health and wellness, social justice, and economic well-being.
- Enhance satisfaction with health care, work, social services, and education.

For practitioners:

- Enhance knowledge.
- Support access to new technology and practices.
- Improve the quality of care or services delivered.
- Improve education.

For institutions:

- Improve quality of leadership.
- Optimize ability to deliver accessible high-quality health care and superior education.
- Acquire ongoing funding.

For the system:

- Expand capacity to provide high-quality health care, social justice, and education.
- Support the efficient provision of care and education.
- Ensure respect for the social, economic, and health care needs of all citizens.

A program's objectives are its specific planned outcomes, to be achieved relatively soon (within six months, a year, three years), although their sustainability can be monitored over time (every year for ten years).

Consider the program objectives in the brief description given in Example 2.2 of an online tutorial.

Example 2.2 The Objectives of a Tutorial to Teach People to Become Savvy Consumers of Online Health Information

Many people go online for information about their health. Research is consistent in finding that online health information varies widely in quality from site to site. In a large city, the Department of Health, Education, and Social Services sponsored the development of a brief online tutorial to assist the community in becoming better consumers of health information [the general, long-range goal]. They conducted focus groups to find out what people wanted to learn and how they like to learn, and they used the findings as well as a model of adult learning to guide the program's instructional features. The evaluators did a preliminary test of the program and found it worked well with the test group.

The tutorial had these three objectives [hoped-for program outcomes for the present time]. At the conclusion of the tutorial, the learner will be able to:

- List at least five criteria for defining the quality of health information.
- Name three high-quality online health information sites.
- Give an unbiased explanation of the symptoms, causes, and treatment of a given health problem using online information.

These objectives became the basis for the evaluation questions, specifically, whether the program is effective in achieving each of the three objectives (Example 2.3).

Example 2.3 Evaluation Questions and Program Objectives

The evaluation team designed a study to find out if an online health information skills tutorial achieved each of its objectives. The team invited people between 20 and 35 years of age who had completed at least two years of university to participate in the evaluation. One group had access to the tutorial, and the other was given a link to a respected site that had a checklist of factors to look for in high-quality health information searches.

The evaluators asked these questions.

1. How did tutorial participants compare to the comparison group on each of the objectives?
2. If the comparisons are in favor of the tutorial group, were they sustained over a 12-month period?

Evaluation Question: How did tutorial participants compare to the control participants on each of the program's objectives?

Hypothesis: The tutorial participants will perform significantly better than the control participants on each objective.

Justification: The research literature suggests that adults learn best if their needs and preferences are respected. This evaluation conducted focus groups to identify needs and preferences. These were incorporated into the tutorial. Also, a model of adult learning guided the program's development. A preliminary test of the program suggested that it would be effective in its targeted population. The comparison group program, although it relied on a well-known and respected site, did not contain incentives to learn.

Study hypotheses are often associated with one or more evaluation questions. A hypothesis is a tentative explanation for an observation, or a scientific problem that can be tested by further investigation. Hypotheses are not arbitrary or based on intuition. They are derived from data collected in previous studies or from a review of the literature. For example, consider this evaluation question, hypothesis, and justification for the evaluation of the online tutorial:

Evaluation questions can be exploratory. Exploratory questions are asked when preliminary data or research is not available to support hypothesis generation. For example, suppose the evaluators of the online tutorial are interested in finding out if differences exist in the achievement of the tutorial's objectives among frequent and infrequent internet users. If no information is available to justify a hypothesis (frequent users will do better), the evaluators can decide to ask an exploratory question, such as "Do frequent internet users learn more than infrequent users?"

Exploratory questions are often interesting and can contribute to new knowledge. However, they also consume resources (time needed for data collection and analysis).

Evaluation Questions: Participants

Evaluation questions often ask about the demographic and social, economic, and health characteristics of the evaluation's participants. The participants include all individuals, institutions, and communities affected by the evaluation's findings. Participation in an evaluation of a school program, for instance, can involve students, teachers, parents, the principal, the school nurse, and representatives of the school's governing boards and local council.

Questions about evaluation participants are illustrated in Example 2.4.

Example 2.4 Evaluation Questions and Participants

The developer of a new program evaluation course for first- and second-year graduate students was concerned with finding out whether the program was effective for all students or only a subset. One measure of effectiveness was the student's ability to prepare a satisfactory evaluation plan. The evaluator asked the following evaluation questions:

- What are the demographic characteristics (age, gender) of each year's students?
- Is the program equally effective for differing students (e.g., males and females)?
- Do first- and second-year students differ in their learning?
- At the end of their second year, did the current first-year students maintain their learning?

Evaluation questions should be answerable with the resources available. Suppose that the evaluation described in Example 2.4 is only a one-year study. In that case, the evaluator cannot answer the question about whether this year's first-year students maintained their learning over the next year. Practical considerations often dampen the ambitions of an evaluation.

Evaluation Questions: Program Characteristics

A program's characteristics include its content, staff, and organization. Example 2.5 gives examples of typical evaluation questions about a program's characteristics.

Example 2.5 Evaluation Questions and Program Characteristics

What is the content of the program? The content includes the topics and concepts that are covered. In an English course, the topics might include writing essays and research papers and naming the parts of a sentence. In a math class, the concepts to cover may include negative and imaginary numbers.

What is the theory or empirical foundation that guides program development? Many programs are built on theories or models of instruction, decision making, or behavior change. Some program developers also rely on previous studies (their own or others') to guide current program development and evaluation.

Who oversees content delivery? Content may be delivered by professionals (teachers, physicians, social workers, nurses) or members of the community (trained peer counselors).

How are the participants "grouped" during delivery? In nearly all evaluations, the program planners or evaluators decide how to assemble participants to deliver the intervention. For instance, in an education program, participants may be in classrooms, the cafeteria, or the gym. In a health setting, participants may attend a clinic or physician's office.

How many sessions or events are to be delivered and for how long? The program may be a ten-minute online weight-loss program that is accessed once a month, a weight-loss app that is accessed on an as-needed basis, or a medically supervised weight-loss program requiring monthly visits to a clinic.

How long does the intervention last? Is it a one-year program? A one-year program in which participants agree to be followed-up for five years?

Evaluation Questions: Financial Costs

Program evaluations can be designed to answer questions about the costs of producing program outcomes. A program's costs consist of any outlay, including money, personnel, time, and facilities (office equipment and buildings). The outcomes may be monetary (numbers of dollars or euros saved) or substantive (years of life saved, or yearly gains in reading or math).

When questions focus on the relationship between costs and monetary outcomes, the evaluation is termed a cost–benefit analysis. When questions are asked about the relationship between costs and substantive outcomes, the evaluation is called a cost-effectiveness analysis. The distinction between evaluations concerned with cost-effectiveness and those addressing cost–benefit is illustrated by these two examples:

- **Cost-effectiveness evaluation:** What are the comparative costs of Programs A and B in providing the means for pregnant women to obtain prenatal care during the first trimester?
- **Cost–benefit evaluation:** For every $100 spent on prenatal care, how many dollars are saved on neonatal intensive care?

Program evaluations tend to pay little attention to questions about costs. Among the reasons are the difficulties inherent in defining costs and measuring benefits and in adding an economic analysis to an already complex evaluation design.

Conducting cost studies requires knowledge of accounting, economics, and statistics. It is often wise to include an economist on the evaluation team if you plan to analyze costs.

Example 2.6 illustrates the types of questions that program evaluators pose about the costs, effects, benefits, and efficiency of health care programs.

Example 2.6 Evaluation Questions: Costs

- What is the relationship between the cost and the effectiveness of three prenatal clinic staffing models: physician-based, mixed staffing, and clinical nurse specialists with physicians available for consultation? Costs include number of personnel, hourly wages, number of prenatal appointments made and kept, and number of hours spent delivering prenatal care. Outcomes include maternal health (such as complications at the time of delivery), neonatal health (such as birth weight), and patient satisfaction.
- How efficient are health care centers' ambulatory clinics? Efficiency is defined as the relationship between the use of practitioner time and the size of a clinic, waiting times for appointments, time spent by faculty in the clinic, and time spent supervising house staff.
- How do the most profitable medical practices differ from the least profitable in terms of types of ownership, collection rates, no-show rates, percentage of patients without insurance coverage, charge for a typical follow-up visit, space occupancy rates, and practitioner costs?
- To what extent does each of three programs to control hypertension produce an annual saving in reduced health care claims that is greater than the annual cost of operating the program? The benefits are costs per hypertensive patient (the costs of operating the program in each year, divided by the number of hypertensive patients being monitored and counseled that year).

Because estimates of program costs are produced over a given two-year period but estimates of savings are produced in a different (later) period, benefits must be adjusted to a standard year. To do this, one must adjust the total claims paid in each calendar year by the consumer price index for medical care costs to a currency standard of a 2024 dollar. The costs of operating the programs are similarly adjusted to 2024 dollars, using the same index.

As these questions illustrate, evaluators must define costs and effectiveness or benefits and, when appropriate, describe the monetary value calculations. Evaluators who answer questions about program costs sometimes perform a *sensitivity analysis* when measures are not precise, or the estimates are uncertain. For example, in a study of the comparative cost-effectiveness of two state-funded school-based health care programs, the evaluators may analyze the influence of increasing each program's funding first by 5% and then by 10% to test the sensitivity of the program's effectiveness to changes in funding level. Through this analysis, the evaluators will be able to tell whether increases in effectiveness keep pace with increases in costs.

Evaluation Questions: The Program's Environment

All programs take place in institutional, social, cultural, and political environments. For instance, Program A, which aims to improve the preventive health care practices of children under age 14, takes place in rural schools and is funded by the national government and the district. Program B has the same aim, but it takes place in a large city and is supported by the city and a private foundation. The social, cultural, and political values of the communities in which the program and the evaluation take place may differ even if the programs have the same aim. It is these values that are likely to influence the choice of evaluation questions and the evidence needed to prove effectiveness, quality, and value.

Environmental matters can get complicated. If an evaluation takes place over several years (say, three years or longer), the social and political context can change. New people and policies may emerge, and these may influence the program and the evaluation. Among the environmental changes that have affected programs in health care, for example, are alterations in reimbursement policies for hospitals and physicians, the development of new technologies, and advances in medical science. In fact, technology, and the need for new types of workers and professionals, has altered the context in which most programs operate.

Evaluation questions about the program's environment are given in Example 2.7.

Example 2.7 Evaluation Questions and the Program's Environment

- **Setting:** Where did the program take place? A school? A clinic? Was the location urban or rural?
- **Funding:** Who funded the program? Government? Non-governmental organization (NGO?) Private foundation? Trust?
- **Managerial structure:** Who is responsible for overseeing the program? Who is responsible and what is the reporting structure? How effective is the managerial structure? If the individuals or groups who are running the program were to leave, would the program continue to be effective?
- **The political context:** Is the political environment (within and outside the institution) supportive of the success of the program? Is the program's support secure?

EVIDENCE OF EFFECTIVENESS, QUALITY, AND VALUE

The evidence used in an evaluation consists of facts and observations that are designed to convince stakeholders that the program's benefits outweigh its risks and costs. For example, consider a program to teach students to conduct evaluations. The program's developers hope to instruct students in many evaluation skills, one of which is how to formulate evaluation questions. The developers also anticipate that the program effects will last over time. The evaluators come up with questions and evidence of a positive outcome:

- **Evaluation question:** Did the program achieve its learning objectives?
- **Evidence:** Of all the students in the new program, 90% will learn to formulate evaluation questions. Learning to formulate questions means identifying and justifying program goals, objectives, and benefits and stating the questions in a comprehensible manner. Evidence that the questions are comprehensible will come from review by at least three potential users of the evaluation.
- **Evaluation question:** Did the program's effects last over time?
- **Evidence:** No decreases in learning will be found between the students' second and first years.

In this case, unless 90% of students learn to formulate questions by the end of the first year and first-year students maintain their learning over a one-year period, the evaluator cannot say the program is effective.

Evidence statements should be specific. The more specific they are, the less likely you will encounter any later disagreement over meaning. Specific evidence (90% of students) is also easier to measure than ambiguous evidence (almost all students).

Ambiguity arises when uniformly accepted definitions or levels of performance are unavailable. For example, in the question "Has the Obstetrical Access and Utilization Initiative improved access to prenatal care for high-risk women?" the terms "improved access to prenatal care" and "high-risk women" are potentially ambiguous. To clarify these terms and thus eliminate ambiguity, the evaluators might find it helpful to engage in a dialogue like the one presented in Example 2.8.

Example 2.8 Clarifying Terms: A Dialogue Between Evaluators

Evaluator 1: "Improved access" means more available and convenient care.

Evaluator 2: What might render care more available and convenient? I did a systematic review of the literature and found that care can be made more available and convenient if some or all the following occur: providing services relatively close to clients' homes; shortening waiting times at clinics; offering financial help; providing assistance with transportation to care; providing aid with child care; and offering education regarding the benefits of prenatal care and compliance with nutrition advice.

Evaluator 1: "High-risk women," according to the Centers for Disease Control, are women whose health and birth outcomes have a higher-than-average chance of being poor. We will need to review the literature to get statistics on average health and birth outcomes.

Evaluator 2: Which, if not all, of the following women will you include? Teens? Users of drugs or alcohol? Smokers? Low-income women? Women with health problems, such as gestational diabetes or hypertension?

The evaluators in Example 2.8 do not arbitrarily clarify the ambiguous terms. Instead, they rely on the research literature and a well-known public health agency for their definitions of improved access and high risk.

The clarification of the question "Has the Obstetrical Access and Utilization Initiative improved access to prenatal care for high-risk women?" is followed by providing evidence of accomplishment as illustrated in Example 2.9.

Example 2.9 Evidence of Access to and Use of Prenatal Care Services

- At least four classes in nutrition and "how to be a parent" will be implemented within three months for teenagers.
- All clinics will provide translation assistance in English, Spanish, Hmong, and Vietnamese within two months.
- Over a five-year period, 80% of all pregnant women without transportation to clinics and community health centers will receive transportation.

A useful way to think about evidence of effectiveness, especially for health care and social welfare programs, is to decide whether you want to focus on structure, process, or outcomes.

The structure of care refers to the environment in which care, including physical and medical health services, is given, as well as the characteristics of the care practitioners (including the number of practitioners and their educational and demographic backgrounds), the setting (e.g., a hospital, prison, school, office, factory, or mental health therapist's office), and the organization of care (how departments and teams are run).

The process of care refers to what is done to and for program participants and includes the procedures, tests, provision of educational materials, and counseling or other therapeutic efforts.

The outcomes of care are the results that come from program participation. These include measures of social, psychological, and physical functioning; satisfaction with care; and quality of life.

Example 2.10 presents illustrative standards for the evaluation question "Has the Obstetrical Access and Utilization Initiative improved access to care for high-risk women?"

Example 2.10 Structure, Process, and Outcome Evidence

- **Structure evidence:** All waiting rooms will have special play areas for patients' children.
- **Process evidence:** All physicians will justify and apply the guidelines prepared by the College of Obstetrics and Gynecology for the number and timing of prenatal care visits to all women.
- **Outcome evidence:** Significantly fewer low-birthweight babies will be born in the experimental group than in the control group, and the difference will be at least as large as the most recent findings reported in the research literature.

Sources of Evidence of Effectiveness, Quality, and Value

How do evaluations decide on the evidence that is acceptable as proof that the program is effective, high quality and of value? There are four possibilities:

1. **Statistical tests:** The evaluation team designs a study in which they compare participants and nonparticipants. If the participants differ statistically from the nonparticipants, and the difference favors participants, the difference constitutes evidence of program success.
2. **Expert advice:** The evaluation team relies on expert advice to set standards of program performance. These individuals, who may include subject matter experts, members of the community, or funding agencies, can help the evaluation team set standards that, based on their experience, are reasonable expectations for program success.
3. **Database consultation:** The evaluation team consults large databases for statistics on educational progress, industry performance, and health behaviors that can be used as benchmarks of program performance.
4. **Literature review:** The evaluation team reviews the research literature to investigate the achievements of similar programs and populations and uses those as evidence of achievement for their program.

Evidence by Comparison: Statistical Significance, Practical Significance, and Effect Size

To obtain statistical evidence, the evaluators compare two or more groups of participants, at least one group of which is in the experimental or new program. If participants in Program A benefit more than participants in Program B do, and the evaluation's design and measures are valid, it may be possible to conclude that Program A is more effective.

It is important to note that just because an evaluation finds statistical differences, and the difference favors participants in the new program, you cannot automatically assume that the new program is effective. At least four questions must be answered before coming to this conclusion.

1. Were the programs comparable to begin with? One program may have better resources or commitment from the staff than the other.
2. Were the participants comparable to begin with? The individuals in one program might be smarter, healthier, more cooperative, or otherwise different from those in the comparison program.
3. Are the measurements valid? Valid measures are accurate and approximate the "truth."
4. Is the magnitude of the difference in outcomes large enough to be meaningful? With very large samples, small differences (e.g., in scores on a standardized test of achievement) can be statistically but not practically or clinically significant. Also, the scale on which the difference is based may not be meaningful. A score of 12 versus a score of 10 is only important if there is research evidence that people with scores of 12 are observably different from people with scores of 10. Are they smarter? Healthier?

Suppose an evaluator is asked to study the effectiveness of an eight-week cognitive-behavioral therapy program for children with measurable symptoms of depression. The evaluation design consists of an experimental group of children who receive the program and a control group of children who do not. In a study design of this type, the participants in the control group may get an alternative program, no program, or they may continue doing what they have been doing all along (usual practice). To guide the evaluation design, the evaluator hypothesizes that the children who make up the two groups are the same in terms of their symptoms before and after the program. This is called the null hypothesis and it can be stated this way: When compared to a control group, children in experimental groups will not differ in their depression scores at the end of the program's eight-week duration.

The evaluator administers standardized measures of depression to all children in both groups before the experimental program begins and then again at the program's conclusion eight weeks later. After analyzing the data using traditional statistical tests, the evaluator finds that the children in the experimental program improved significantly in their scores on the depression measure when compared to children in the control group. Using these statistical findings, the evaluator rejects the hypothesis that the two groups are the same after the program is completed and concludes that because the groups differ statistically, the program is effective.

Some of the children's teachers challenge the evaluator's conclusion by asking if the statistical difference is meaningful in practice. The teachers are not convinced that the experimental group's improvement in scores means much. After all, they argue, the depression measure is not perfect, the difference in scores was not that large, and the measured gains may disappear over time.

Through this experience, the evaluator learns that if you rely solely on statistical significance as evidence of effectiveness, you may be challenged to prove that the statistics mean something practical and enduring.

Assume that students' scores on a standardized test of achievement increase from 150 to 160. Does this ten-point increase mean that students are more capable? How much money are policy makers willing to allocate for schools to improve scores by ten points?

Consider a group of people in which each loses ten pounds after being on a diet for six months. Depending on where each person started (some may need to lose no more than ten pounds, but some may need to lose 50), a loss of ten pounds may be clinically significant. Practical significance is linked to program value because unless the magnitude of the outcomes is meaningful to potential users (like people trying to lose weight), policy makers may decide the costs of the program outweigh the relatively small benefits.

Another way to think of evidence of practical significance is through the concept of effect size. Consider this conversation between two evaluators:

Evaluator A: We have been asked to evaluate a web-based program for high school students whose aim is to decrease their risky behaviors (such as drinking and driving; smoking) through interactive education and the use of online support groups. We particularly want students to stop smoking. How will we know if the program is effective? Has anyone done a study like this?

Evaluator B: I don't know of anyone offhand, but we can contact some people I know who have worked extensively to study online programs to reduce health risks. Maybe they have some data we can use. Also, we can do a search of the literature.

Evaluator A: What do we look for?

Evaluator B: Programs with evidence of statistically significant reductions in proportions of students who smoke and drink. Once we find them, we will have to decide if the reduction is large enough to be clinically as well as statistically meaningful for our students. What proportion of teens in each program need to quit smoking or drinking will convince stakeholders and policy makers that our program is effective and has value? For instance, if 10% of teens quit, is that good enough, or do we expect to see 15% or even 20%?

Evaluator B is getting at the concept of effect size when she talks about observing a sufficiently large number of students who quit smoking or drinking so that the outcome, if statistically significant, is also clinically significant.

Effect size is a way of quantifying the size of the difference between two groups. It places the emphasis on the most important aspect of a program—the size of the effect—rather than its statistical significance. The difference between statistical significance and effect as evidence of effectiveness is illustrated by these two questions:

Question 1: Does participation in Program A result in a smaller percentage of smokers than Program B, and when using standard statistical tests, is the difference significant? Any reduction in percentage is acceptable if the difference is statistically significant.

Question 2: Does Program A result in 25% fewer smokers or an even greater reduction [effect] than Program B? Anything less than 25% is not clinically important even if it is statistically significant.

How do you determine a desirable effect size? As Evaluator B (above) suggests, one source of information is data from other programs. Previously collected data provides a guide to the accomplishments of other programs. Evaluators must then decide if the accomplishments are appropriate based on whether the participants and resources used in both programs are alike.

In some cases, data is not available, as is likely to happen when the program you are evaluating is relatively innovative in design or objectives. Without existing data, you may have to conduct a small-scale or pilot study to get estimates of effect sizes that you can reasonably aim for in your evaluation.

A typical effect size calculation considers the standardized mean (average) difference between two groups. In other words:

$$\text{Effect Size} = \frac{[\text{Mean of experimental group}] - [\text{Mean of control group}]}{\text{Standard Deviation}}$$

A rule of thumb for interpreting effect sizes is that a "small" effect size is .20, a "medium" effect size is .50, and a "large" effect size is .80. However, not only do evaluators want to be sure that the effect is meaningful, but they also want to be certain they have a large enough number of people in their study to detect a meaningful effect if one exists. The technique for determining sample sizes to detect an effect of a given size (small, medium, or large) is called power analysis (see Chapter 4).

Evidence from Expert Consultation: Professionals, Consumers, Community Groups

Experts can assist evaluators in deciding on evidence and in confirming the practical or clinical significance of the findings. An expert is any individual or group that is likely to use or has an interest in the results of an evaluation.

Evaluators use a variety of techniques to consult with and promote agreement among experts. These usually include selecting representative groups of people who are experienced in the discipline addressed by the program and bringing them together in a formalized manner.

The fields of public health and medicine make extensive use of experts. For example, the U.S. National Institutes of Health has convened expert consensus development conferences for decades to resolve issues related to knowledge about and use of medical technologies, such as intraocular lens implantation, as well as to the care of patients with specific conditions, such as depression, sleep disorders, traveler's diarrhea, and breast cancer.

The use of experts has proven to be an effective technique in program evaluation for setting evidence of performance, as illustrated in Example 2.11.

Example 2.11 Using Experts to Decide on Evidence

Sixteen U.S. teaching hospitals participated in a four-year evaluation of a program to improve outpatient care in their group practices. Among the study's major goals were improvements in the amount of faculty involvement in the practices, in staff productivity, and in access to care for patients. The evaluators and representatives from each of the hospitals used evidence for care established by the Institute of Medicine as a basis for setting evidence of program effectiveness before the start of the study. After two years, the evaluators presented interim data on performance and brought experts from the 16 hospitals together to come to consensus on evidence for the final two years of the study. To guide the process, the evaluators prepared a special form, a portion of which appears in Table 2.1.

Guidelines for Expert Panels

Following a few simple instructions can assist evaluators in the effective use of expert panels in identifying evaluation evidence.

1. Evaluation questions must be unambiguous. Unambiguous questions define the independent and dependent or outcome variables and leave little room for disagreement among panelists.

Compare Questions A and B.

A. **Not quite ready for evidence-setting:** Was the program effective with high-risk women?

This question is ambiguous because the terms "effective" (dependent variable) and "high-risk" (independent variable) can be interpreted in many ways.

B. **Ready for evidence-setting:** When compared to a control group, did the program improve the proportion of low-weight births among low-income women?

Table 2.1 Selected Portion of a Form Used to Decide on Evaluation Program Evidence

Variable	Current Evidence	Definitions	Interim Results	Question	Our View	Your Decision
Waiting Time	90% of patients should be seen within 30 minutes	Waiting time is time between scheduled appointment and when first seen by primary provider	70% of patients were seen within 30 minutes	Is 90% reasonable?	90%	%
	Compared to national databases, program patients should not have unduly long waiting times		Waiting times = 24.3 minutes National data = 37.3 minutes for doctor's office or private clinic	Should national data be used as evidence?	Yes	Yes No

This question is not ambiguous. The dependent variable is low birthweight, and the independent variable is low-income women (because the literature provides evidence that income is related to risk in pregnancy with lower-income women at greater risk). Both low birthweight and low income must be defined. Fortunately, standard measures exist for each concept. The dependent variable and hoped-for outcome or evidence of effectiveness is a statistically observed improvement in the proportion of low-weight births among women who participate in the experimental program when compared to a control.

2. The evaluator should provide the experts with data to help in decision making. The data can be about the participants in the experimental program, the program itself, and the costs and benefits of participation. The data can come from published literature, from ongoing research, or from financial and statistical records. For example, in an evaluation of a program to improve birthweight among infants born to low-income women, experts' decision making might be made easier if they have information about the extent of the problem in the country. They might also want to know how prevalent low-weight births are among poor women, and if other interventions have been used effectively, what their costs were.

3. The evaluator should select experts based on their knowledge and influence. The number of experts an evaluator chooses is necessarily dependent on the evaluation's resources and the evaluator's skill in coordinating groups. (See Example 2.12 for two illustrations concerning the choice of experts.)

Example 2.12 Choosing Experts to Guide the Choice of Evaluation Evidence

- The New Dental Clinic wants to improve patient satisfaction. A meeting was held during which three patient representatives, including a nurse, a physician, and a technician, defined the "satisfied patient" and decided on how much time to allow the clinic to produce satisfied patients.
- The primary goals of the Adolescent Outreach Program are to teach young people about preventive health care and to make sure that all needed health care services (such as vision screening and immunizations) are provided to them. A group of young people participated in a teleconference to help the program developers and evaluators decide on the best ways to teach teens and to set evidence of learning achievement. Also, physicians, social workers, nurses, teachers, and parents participated in a conference to determine the types of services that should be provided and how many teens should receive them annually.

---

4. The evaluator should ensure that the panel process is carefully structured and skillfully led. A major purpose of the expert panel is to come to agreement on the criteria for appraising a program's performance. To facilitate agreement, and to distinguish the panel process from an open-ended committee meeting, the evaluator should prepare an agenda for the panel in advance, along with the other materials such as literature reviews and other presentations of data. The panel's tasks must be specific, and the panel leader should be experienced in and comfortable with large groups of people who will inevitably have diverse perspectives.

Evidence from Existing Data and Large Databases

Large databases, such as those maintained by the U.S. Centers for Disease Control and Prevention (CDC) and other nations through their government agencies and registries, come from surveys of whole populations and contain information on individual and collective health, education, and social functioning. The rules and regulations for gaining access to these databases vary. Some evaluators also compile their own data sets, and some make them available to other investigators.

The information in large databases (and their summaries and reports) can provide benchmarks against which evaluators can measure the effectiveness of new programs. For instance, an evaluator of a hypothetical drivers' education program might say something like this: "I used the province's Surveillance Data Set to find out about the use of seat belts. The results show that in this province, about five out of ten drivers between the ages of 18 and 21 years do not use seat belts. An effective driver education program should be able to improve on that number to reduce it to two drivers out of ten within five years."

Suppose you were asked to evaluate a new program to prevent low-weight births in your province region. If you know the current percentage of low-weight births in the province, then you can use that figure as a benchmark for evaluating the effectiveness of a new program that aims to lower the rate. Example 2.13 illustrates how evaluators use existing data as evidence of effectiveness.

Example 2.13 Using Existing Data as Evidence

- The Obstetrical Access and Utilization Initiative serves high-risk women and aims to reduce the numbers of births of babies weighing less than 2,500 grams (5.5 pounds). One evaluation question asks, "Is the birth of low-weight babies prevented?" In the state, 6.1% of babies are low birthweight, but this percentage includes babies born to women who are at low or medium risk. The evidence used as proof that low-weight births are prevented is as follows: "No more than 6.1% of babies will be born weighing less than 5.5 pounds."
- The city's governing council decides that the schools should become partners with the community's health care clinics in developing and evaluating a program to reduce motor vehicle crashes among young adults between the ages 18 to 24 years. According to the Centers for Disease Control's findings from the Youth Risk Behavior Surveillance System, the leading cause of death (31% of all deaths) among youth of this age is motor vehicle accidents.
- Council members, community clinic representatives, teachers and administrators from the schools, and young people meet to discuss evidence of program effectiveness. They agree that they would like to see a statistically and clinically meaningful reduction in deaths due to motor vehicle crashes over the program's five-year trial period. They use the 31% figure as the baseline against which to evaluate any reduction.

When you use data from large databases as evidence of a local program's effectiveness, you must make certain that the data is applicable to the current local setting. The only data available to you may have been collected a long time ago or under circumstances that are very different from those surrounding the program you are evaluating, and so they may not apply. For example, data collected from an evaluation conducted with men may not apply to women, and data on older men may not apply to younger men. Data collected ten years ago may now be obsolete because the population in the community has changed since then.

Evidence from the Research Literature

The research literature consists of all peer-reviewed evaluation reports. Most, not all, of these reports are either published or expected to be published. Evaluators should use only the most scientifically rigorous evaluations as the basis for applying evidence of effectiveness, quality, and value from one program to another. They must be careful to check that the evaluated program included participants and settings that are similar to those in the new program. Example 2.14 illustrates how evaluators can use the literature in setting evidence in program evaluations.

Example 2.14 Using the Literature to Find and Justify Effectiveness Evaluation Evidence

The Community Cancer Center has inaugurated a new program to help families deal with the depressive symptoms that often accompany a diagnosis of cancer in a loved one. The main program objective is to reduce symptoms of depression among participating family members.

The evaluators want to convene a group of potential program participants to assist in developing evidence of program effectiveness. Specifically, the evaluators want assistance in defining "reduction in symptoms." They discover, however, that is it nearly impossible to find a mutually convenient time for a meeting with potential participants. Also, the Center does not have the funds to sponsor a face-to-face meeting. Because of these constraints, the evaluators decide against a meeting and instead turn to the literature.

The evaluators go online to find research articles that describe the effectiveness of programs to reduce depressive symptoms in cancer patients. Although they find five published articles, only one of the programs has the same objectives and similar participants as the Community Cancer Center's program, and it took place in an academic cancer center. Nevertheless, given the quality of the evaluation and the similarities in the two programs' objectives, the evaluators believe that they can apply the other program's evidence to the present program. This is what the evaluators found in the article:

> At the six-month assessment period, family members in the first group had significantly lower self-reported symptoms of depression on the Depression Scale than did family members in the second group (8.9 versus 15.5). The mean difference between groups adjusted for baseline scores was -7.0 (95% confidence interval, -10.8 to -3.2), an effect size of 1.08 standard deviations. These results suggest that 86% of those who underwent the program reported lower scores of depressive symptoms at six months than would have been expected if they had not undergone the program.

The evaluators decide to use the same measure of depressive symptoms (the Depression Scale) as evaluator of the published study and to use the same statistical test to determine the significance of the results.

When adopting evidence from the literature, you must compare the characteristics of the program you are evaluating and the program or programs whose evaluation evidence you plan to adopt. You need to make certain that the participants, settings, interventions, and primary outcomes are demonstrably similar between the two. Then, when you conduct your evaluation, you must choose the same measures or instruments and statistical methods.

WHEN TO DECIDE ON EVIDENCE OF EFFECTIVENESS, QUALITY, AND VALUE

The evaluation should have evidence of effectiveness in place *before* continuing with design and analysis. Evidence of effectiveness guides the evaluation's design, data collection, and analysis, and choosing it in advance is the only way to prevent bias.

Consider the following two examples.

Example 1

- *Program goal*: To teach research assistants to reliably extract data from medical databases.
- *Evaluation question*: Have assistants learned to reliably extract data from medical databases?
- *Evidence*: 90% of all assistants reliably extract data from medical databases.

- *Program effects on*: Assistants.
- *Effects measured by*: Extent to which extractions result in reliable data.
- *Design*: Observational survey design.
- *Data collection*: Two experts review a sample of extractions.
- *Statistical analysis*: Extent to which the experts statistically agree (use of the *kappa* statistic) on the reliability of the assistants' extractions.

Example 2

- *Program goal*: To teach research assistants to reliably extract data from medical databases.
- *Evaluation question*: Have assistants learned to reliably extract data from medical databases?
- *Evidence*: A statistically significant difference in learning is observed between assistants at Medical Center A and assistants at Medical Center B. Assistants at Medical Center A participated in a new program, and the difference is in their favor.
- *Program effects on*: Assistants at Medical Center A.
- *Effects measured by*: Extent to which data from extractions is reliable.
- *Design*: A comparison of two groups of assistants.
- *Data collection*: A test of the assistants' ability to extract data. The test yields scores of 10 to 100, with 100 equaling perfect reliability.
- *Statistical Analysis*: A *t*-test to compare average abstractions scores between assistants at Medical Center A and assistants at Medical Center B.

As can be seen from the examples, the evidence dictates the program's design (observational versus comparison), the data collection methods (agreement by experts), and the statistical methods (kappa versus *t*-test).

The evaluation questions and evidence contain within them the independent and dependent variables on which the evaluation's design, measurement, and analysis are subsequently based. Independent variables are sometimes called explanatory or predictor variables because they are present before the start of the program (i.e., they are independent of it).

Evaluators use independent variables to explain or predict outcomes. In the example above, reliable extraction of medical data (the outcome) is to be explained by nurses' participation in a new program (the independent variable). In evaluations, the independent variables often are the program (experimental and control), demographic features of the participants (such as gender, income, education, experience), and other characteristics of the participants that might affect outcomes (such as physical, mental, and social health; knowledge).

Dependent variables, also termed outcome variables, are the factors the evaluator expects to measure because they are the program's results. In program evaluations, outcome variables include knowledge, skills, attitudes, behaviors, health and well-being, living status, costs, and efficiency.

The evaluation questions and evidence necessarily contain the independent and dependent variables within them as illustrated in Example 2.15.

Example 2.15 Questions, Evidence, and Independent and Dependent Variables

Program goal: To teach research assistants to extract reliable data from medical databases.
Evaluation question: Have assistants learned to reliably extract data from medical database.
Evidence: A statistically significant difference in learning is observed between assistants at Medical Center A and assistants at Medical Center B. Assistants at Medical Center A participated in a new program, and the difference is in their favor.
Independent variable: Participation versus no participation in a new program.
Dependent variable or what will be measured at end of program participation: Reliable data extraction.

PROGRAM EVALUATION AND ECONOMICS

In recent years, it has become increasingly important that evaluators provide evidence to stakeholders that a program is effective, has value, and is worth financial investment.

Program evaluations use four types of cost analysis to investigate and provide evidence of a program's value.

Cost Analysis to Investigate and Provide Evidence of a Program's Value

- **Cost-effectiveness evaluation:** Program A is effective if it is less costly than any other effective program.
- **Cost–benefit analysis:** Program A has merit if its benefits are equal to or exceed its costs; the benefit-to-cost ratio of Program A is equal to or greater than 1.0 and exceeds the benefit-to-cost ratio of Program B.
- **Cost minimization analysis:** Programs A and B have identical benefits, but Program A has lower costs.
- **Cost utility analysis:** Program A produces N (the evaluation figures out exactly how many) quality-adjusted life years at lower cost than Program B. The quality-adjusted life year (QALY) is a measure of disease burden, including both the quality and the quantity of life lived. It is used in assessing the value for money of a medical intervention. The QALY is based on the number of years of life that would be added by the intervention.

Example 2.16 illustrates the uses of economic evidence in evaluations.

Example 2.16 Evidence Used in Economic Evaluations

RISK-FREE is a new anti-smoking program. The evaluators have three study aims and associated hypotheses. Two of the study aims (Aims 2 and 3) pertain to an economic evaluation.

Aim 1: To evaluate the comparative effectiveness of an app to prevent smoking in young adults relative to the current program, which consists of lectures, videos, and discussion.

Hypothesis 1: When baseline levels are controlled for, the experimental students (using the app) will have a significantly lower probability of starting to smoke over a 12-month period than students in the current program.

Hypothesis 2: When baseline levels are controlled for, the experimental students will have significantly better quality of life over a 12-month period than students in the current program.

Hypothesis 3: When baseline levels are controlled for, the experimental students will demonstrate significantly greater self-efficacy and knowledge over a 12-month period than students in the current program.

Hypothesis 4: When baseline levels are controlled for, the experimental teachers will demonstrate significantly greater knowledge and more positive attitudes than teachers in the current program.

Aim 2: To evaluate the comparative costs of the app relative to the current program.

Hypothesis 5: When baseline levels are controlled for, the experimental students will have significantly lower need for counseling and net (intervention plus nonintervention) costs over a 12-month period than students in the current program.

Aim 3: To evaluate the cost-effectiveness of the app relative to the current program.

Hypothesis 6: The experimental app will be cost-effective relative to the current program, based on generally accepted threshold values for incremental cost-effectiveness ratios.

If Aim 2 demonstrates that the program is cost saving because it has equal outcomes or is cost neutral because it has better outcomes, then the app is cost-effective, and the Aim 3 analyses are unnecessary.

THE QEV REPORT: QUESTIONS, EVIDENCE, VARIABLES

The relationships among evaluation questions, evidence, and outcome variables can be depicted in a reporting form like the one in Table 2.2. As you can see the evaluation questions appear in the first column of the QEV (questions, evidence, variables) report form, followed in subsequent columns by the evidence associated with each question, the independent variables, and the dependent variables.

The QEV report in Table 2.2 shows information on an evaluation of an 18-month program combining diet and exercise to improve health status and quality of life for people

Table 2.2 A Report to Describe the Evaluation Questions, Evidence, and the Outcome Variables

Evaluation Questions	Evaluation Evidence	Independent or Explanatory Variables	Dependent or Outcome Variables
Has the new program achieved its objectives? Objective 1: To what extent has quality of life improved?	A statistically and practically significant improvement in quality of life over a one-year period. A statistically and practically significant improvement in quality of life between participants and nonparticipants	Gender, program participation (experimental and control participants), patient mix (demographic characteristics, functional status scores, presence of chronic disorders, such as diabetes and hypertension)	Quality of life includes social contacts and support, financial support, perceptions of well-being
Has the new program achieved its objectives? Objective 2: To what extent has health status improved?	A statistically and practically significant improvement in quality of life over a one-year period. A statistically and practically significant improvement in quality of life between participants and nonparticipants	Gender, program participation, (experimental and control participants), and patient mix (demographic characteristics, functional status scores, presence of chronic disorders, such as diabetes and hypertension)	Health status includes functional status and perceptions of general health and physical functioning; measures of complications from illness (for diabetes complications include cardiac, renal, ophthalmologic, or foot) for hypertension complications include poor blood pressure control)
What is the relationship between cost and effectiveness of two clinic staffing models: primarily physicians and primarily nurses?	Effectiveness will be demonstrated by lower cost per visit, satisfactory health status, and satisfactory quality of life	Two models of care (primarily physician-based and primarily nurse-based)	Quality of life, health status, costs of personnel, hours delivering care, number of appointments made and kept

75 years of age or older who are living at home. Participants will be randomly assigned to the experimental or control groups according to the streets where they live. Participants in the evaluation who need medical services can choose one of two clinics offering differing models of care delivery, one that is primarily staffed by physicians and one that is primarily staffed by nurses.

The evaluators will be investigating whether any differences exist between male and female participants after program participation and the role of patient mix in those differences. (*Patient mix* refers to the characteristics of patients that might affect the dependent variables or outcomes. The dependent variables in this evaluation include demographic characteristics, functional status scores, and presence of chronic disorders such as diabetes and hypertension.) The evaluators will also be analyzing the cost-effectiveness of the two models of health care delivery.

This evaluation has three questions: one about the program's influence on quality of life, one about the program's influence on health status, and one about the cost-effectiveness of two methods for staffing clinics. Each of the three questions has one or more types of evidence associated with it. The independent variables for the questions about quality of life and health status are gender, group participation, and patient mix, and each of these terms is explained. The dependent or outcome variables are also explained in the QEV report. For example, the report notes that "quality of life" includes social contacts and support, financial support, and perceptions of well-being.

SUMMARY AND TRANSITION TO THE NEXT CHAPTER ON DESIGNING PROGRAM EVALUATIONS

A program evaluation is conducted to determine whether unbiased evidence exists to demonstrate that a program is effective and has high quality and value. Is the program worth its costs, or will a more efficient program accomplish even more? Evaluation questions are the evaluation's centerpiece. Their combined answers provide evidence about the extent to which program goals and objectives have been met and the degree, duration, costs, and distribution of benefits and harms. The evaluation questions can also ask about the program's social and political environment and the implementation and effectiveness of different program activities and management strategies. Selecting and justifying evaluation questions means weighing the importance of the questions against the evaluation's resources.

The evaluator must decide on the questions or hypotheses and evidence in advance of any evaluation activities because both together prescribe the evaluation's design, data collection, and analysis. Evaluation evidence comes from comparing other programs, from the opinions of experts, and from reviews of the literature and existing databases.

The next chapter tells you how to design an evaluation so that you will be able to link any changes found in knowledge, attitudes, and behaviors to a new or experimental program and not to other competing events. For example, suppose you are evaluating a school campaign that aims to encourage high school students to drink water instead of energy drinks. You might conclude that your program is effective because you observed a significant increase in water-drinking among program participants. However, if your evaluation's design is not sufficiently robust to distinguish between the effects of the program and other sources of education, such as social media and television, then your conclusion might be incorrect. The next chapter discusses evaluation designs and provides guidance for conducting rigorous evaluations.

EXERCISES: CHAPTER 2

Directions

Read the evaluation descriptions below, and, using the information offered, list the evaluation questions; associated evidence of program effectiveness, quality, and value; and the independent and dependent variables.

1. Gambling and College Students

College students experience high rates of problem and pathological gambling, yet little research has investigated methods for reducing gambling in this population. This study sought to examine the effectiveness of brief intervention strategies. Seventeen college students were assigned randomly to an assessment-only control, ten minutes of brief advice, one session of motivational enhancement therapy (MET), or one session of MET plus three sessions of cognitive-behavioral therapy (CBT). The three interventions were designed to reduce gambling. Gambling was assessed at baseline, after six weeks, and at the ninth month using the Addiction Severity Index–gambling (ASI-G) module, which also assesses days and dollars wagered.

2. Drug Education and Elementary School

The evaluators conducted a short-term evaluation of the Always Be Careful (ABC) program which aims to prevent drug abuse among students in primary school and keep them in school. The evaluators examined the program's effects on students' 30-day use of tobacco, alcohol, and marijuana, as well as on their school attendance. The evaluation included students in 17 urban schools, each of which served as its own control. Fifth graders in the 2023–2024 school year constituted the comparison group (n = 1490), and those enrolled as 5th graders in the 2024–2025 school year constituted the ABC intervention group (n = 1450). The evaluators found no intervention effect on students' substance use for any of the substance use outcomes assessed. They did find that students were more likely to attend school on days they received ABC program lessons, but they also found that students in the ABC group were more likely to have been suspended. The evaluators concluded that the evidence did not support implementation and dissemination of the ABC program.

REFERENCES AND SUGGESTED READINGS

Campos, L., Dias, P., Duarte, A., Veiga, E., Dias, C.C., & Palha F. (2018). Is it possible to "Find Space for Mental Health" in young people? Effectiveness of a school-based mental health literacy promotion program. *International Journal of Environmental Research and Public Health, 15*(7): 1426.

Coulton, S., Stockdale, K., Marchand, C., et al. (2017). Pragmatic randomised controlled trial to evaluate the effectiveness and cost effectiveness of a multi-component intervention to reduce substance use and risk-taking behaviour in adolescents involved in the criminal justice system: A trial protocol (RISKIT-CJS). *BMC Public Health, 17*(1): 246.

Gillam, S.L, Vaughn, S., Roberts, G., et al. (2023). Improving oral and written narration and reading comprehension of children at-risk for language and literacy difficulties: Results of a randomized clinical trial. *Journal of Educational Psychology, 115*: 99–117.

Katz, C., Bolton, S.L., Katz, L.Y., Isaak, C., Tilston-Jones, T., & Sareen. J. (2013). A systematic review of school-based suicide prevention programs. Depression and Anxiety, *30*(10): 1030–1045.

Krebs, E. & Nosyk, B. (2021). Cost-effectiveness analysis in implementation science: A research agenda and call for wider application. *Current HIV/AIDS Reports, 18*(3): 176–185.

Moodie, M.L., Herbert, J.K., de Silva-Sanigorski, A.M., et al. (2013). The cost-effectiveness of a successful community-based obesity prevention program: The Be Active Eat Well program. *Obesity, 21*(10): 2072–2080.

Ruiz-Casares, M., Thombs, B.D., Mayo, N.E., Andrina, M., Scott, S.C., & Platt, R.W. (2022). The Families First Program to prevent child abuse: Results of cluster randomized controlled trial in West Java, Indonesia. *Prevention Science*, 23(8): 1457–1469.

Suggested Websites

The CDC's evaluation framework and guidelines
www.cdc.gov/evaluation/index.htm

Wikipedia for Cost Analyses
https://en.wikipedia.org/wiki/Cost-effectiveness_analysis

ANSWERS TO THE EXERCISES: CHAPTER 2

Exercise 1

Evaluation question: Did the program (brief intervention) achieve its objective of reducing gambling?

Evidence: A reduction in gambling at week six and month nine.

Independent variable: Program participation (assessment-only control, ten minutes of brief advice, one session of motivational enhancement therapy (MET) or one session of MET plus three sessions of cognitive-behavioral therapy (CBT)).

Dependent variable: Reduction in gambling as measured by the Addiction Severity Index (ASI-G) module, which also assesses days and dollars wagered.

Exercise 2

Evaluation question: Did the revised curriculum achieve beneficial outcomes? The outcomes of interest include tobacco, alcohol, and marijuana use; school attendance.

Evidence: Implied: decreased use of tobacco, alcohol, and marijuana; improvements in attendance.

Independent variable: Program participation (2022–2023, 5th graders) = comparison group; (2023–2024, 5th graders) = revised curriculum group).

Dependent variables: Substance use; attendance.

CHAPTER 3 | DESIGNING PROGRAM EVALUATIONS

An evaluation's design is its unique research structure. The structure has five components:

1. Evaluation questions and hypotheses.
2. Evidence of effectiveness, quality, value.
3. Criteria for study eligibility.
4. Rules for assigning participants to programs.
5. Rules for the timing and frequency of data collection or measurement.

Each of these design components is discussed in detail in this chapter. The chapter also explains the uses and limitations of experimental (randomized controlled trials and nonrandomized controlled trials or quasi-experiments) and observational (cohorts, case control, cross-sectional) evaluation designs. In addition, the chapter explains how to minimize research design bias through blocking, stratification, and blinding.

The chapter also discusses and explains factorial, non-inferiority, and comparative effectiveness research (CER). In the real world, evaluators must deal with practical and methodological challenges that prevent them from conducting the perfect study. These challenges, if not confronted head-on, may "threaten" or bias the evaluation's validity. This chapter discusses the most typical threats to an evaluation design's internal and external validity and explains how to guard against these threats using statistical and other more field-friendly techniques.

A READER'S GUIDE TO CHAPTER 3

Evaluation Design: Creating the Structure
Experimental Evaluation Designs
    The Randomized Controlled Trial or RCT
    Parallel Controls
    Waitlist Controls
Randomizing and Blinding
    Random Assignment
    Random Clusters
    Improving on Chance: Stratifying and Blocking
    Blinding

DOI: 10.4324/9781032635071-3

EVALUATION DESIGN: CREATING THE STRUCTURE

An evaluation design is a structure that is created specially to produce unbiased information about a program's effectiveness, quality, and value. Biases in evaluations lead to systematic errors in the findings. They can occur at any stage of the evaluation, but flawed research designs are very common causes.

An evaluation's design has five structural components:

1. Evaluation questions and hypotheses.
2. Anticipated evidence of effectiveness, quality, value.
3. Criteria for study eligibility.
4. Rules for assigning participants to programs.
5. Rules for the timing and frequency of measurement.

Example 3.1 describes three basic evaluation designs. As you can see, the designs are applied to an evaluation of the same program and have the same structural components. However, there are differences between the designs. The main difference between Design 1 and Design 2 is in the way that the schools are assigned: at *random* or not at random. Random assignment means that all experimental *units* (schools in this case) have an equal chance of being in the experimental or control program. The main difference between both Designs 1 and 2 and Design 3 is that in Design 3, the evaluator uses data from an already existing program database: no new data is collected, and assignment is not an issue.

Example 3.1 Three Basic Evaluation Designs for One Program: Spanish-Language Health Education for Fifth Graders

Program: A new Spanish-language health education program for fifth graders is being evaluated in six of the district's elementary schools. If effective, it will be introduced throughout the district. Three of the schools will continue with their regular English-language health education program, and the other three will participate in the new program. The main program objective is to improve students' knowledge of nutrition. The program developers anticipate that the new program will be more effective in improving this knowledge.

The evaluators will use statistical techniques to test the hypothesis that no differences in knowledge will be found. They hope to prove that assumption to be false. Students will be given a knowledge test within one month of the beginning of the program and after one year to determine how much they have learned.

1. Experimental Evaluation Design with Random Assignment

Evaluation question: Does the program achieve its objective?
Hypothesis: No differences will be found in knowledge between students in the new and standard program over a one-year period.
Evidence: Statistically significant improvement over time favoring the new program (rejecting the hypothesis that no differences exist).
Eligibility: Students who read at the fifth-grade level or better in Spanish.
Assignment to programs: Using a computer-generated program of random numbers, five schools are randomly assigned to the new program and five to the standard program.
Measurement frequency and timing: A test of students' knowledge within one month of the beginning of the program and a test of students' knowledge one year after completion of the program

2. Experimental Evaluation Design Without Random Assignment

Evaluation question: Does the program achieve its objective?
Hypothesis: No differences will be found in knowledge between students in the new and standard program.
Evidence: Statistically significant improvement over time favoring the new program (rejecting the hypothesis that no differences exist) over a one-year period.
Eligibility: Students who read at the fifth-grade level or better in Spanish.
Assignment to programs: Evaluators create five pairs of schools with schools in each pair matched so that they have similar student demographics and resources. Using a computer-generated table of random numbers, one of each pair of schools is assigned to the new or standard program resulting in five schools in the experimental group and five in the control group.
Measurement frequency and timing: A test of students' knowledge within one month of the beginning of the program, and a test of students' knowledge one year after completion of the program.

3. Observational Evaluation Design

Evaluation question: Does the program achieve its objective?
Hypothesis: No differences will be found in knowledge between students in the new and standard program.
Evidence: Statistically significant improvement over time favoring the new program (rejecting the hypothesis that no differences exist) over a one-year period.
Eligibility: Students who read at the fifth-grade level or better in Spanish.
Assignment to programs: The evaluation occurs after the program has already been completed, and all data has been entered into the program's database. The evaluators develop an algorithm to identify which students were in the experimental and which were in the comparison group. They also use the algorithm to identify the students who provided complete knowledge test data. Not all students will have completed all tests; some may have completed only parts of each test.
Measurement frequency and timing: The evaluators were not consulted on measurement policy. With luck, the program team administered knowledge tests at regular intervals and large numbers of students completed all tests with few unanswered questions.

Example 3.1 illustrates three basic program evaluation designs: (1) experimental evaluation designs *with* random assignment into experimental and control programs (the randomized controlled trial or RCT), (2) experimental evaluation designs *without* random assignment into programs, and (3) observational evaluation designs that use existing data on programs regardless of how participants were assigned.

Random assignment is a method that relies on the unpredictable, or *chance*, to assign participants to programs. Suppose the evaluation aims to compare how well people in Program A learn when compared to people in Program B. With random assignment, every eligible person has an equal chance of ending up in one of the two programs. The assignment takes place by using a random numbers table or a computer-generated random sequence of numbers (found in statistical programs and online).

A nonrandomized or quasi-experimental evaluation design is one in which experimental and comparison groups are created without random assignment. In the second illustration in Example 3.1, the schools are matched according to preset criteria, such as demographics and resources, and then randomly assigned to programs. Matching is just one way of creating groups for nonrandomized trials.

Other nonrandomization options include allocating participants to programs by their date of birth, or medical or school record number, or assigning every other person on a list of eligible participants to the new or comparison program. Nonrandom assignment does not ensure that participants have an equal chance of receiving the experimental or comparison programs.

Randomized and nonrandomized controlled trials are frequently contrasted with observational evaluation designs. *Observational* or *descriptive designs* are different from controlled trials because the evaluation is conducted using an existing database: no new data is collected. In the third illustration in Example 3.1, the evaluators do their analysis after all program data has been collected; they have no say about assignment to programs.

EXPERIMENTAL EVALUATION DESIGNS

The Randomized Controlled Trial or RCT

An RCT is an experimental evaluation design in which eligible individuals (doctors, prison guards, lawyers, students) or groups (schools, prisons, hospitals, communities) are assigned at random to one of several programs or interventions.

The RCT is considered the gold standard of designs because, when implemented properly, it can be counted on to rule out inherent participant characteristics that may affect the program's outcomes. Put another way, if participants are assigned to experimental and control programs randomly, then the two groups will probably be alike in all important ways before they participate. If they are different afterwards, the difference can be reasonably linked to the program. If the evaluation design is robust, it may be possible to say that the program caused the outcome.

Suppose the evaluators of a health literacy program in the workplace hope to improve employees' writing skills. They recruit volunteers to participate in a six-week writing program and compare their writing skills to those of other workers who are, on average, the same age and have similar educational backgrounds and writing skills. Also, suppose that after the volunteers complete the six-week program, the evaluators compare the writing of the two groups and find that the experimental group performs much better.

Can the evaluators claim that the literacy program is effective? Possibly. But the nature of the design is such that you cannot really tell if some other factors that the evaluators did not measure are the ones that are responsible for the apparent program success. The volunteers may have done better because they were more motivated to achieve (that is why they volunteered), have more home-based social support, and so on.

A better way to evaluate the workplace literacy program is to (1) randomly assign all eligible workers (e.g., those who score below a certain level on a writing test) to the experimental program or to a comparable control program, and (2) then compare changes in writing skills over time. With random assignment, all the important factors (such as motivation and home support) are likely to be equally distributed between the two groups. Then, if writing test scores are significantly different after the evaluation is concluded, and the scores favor the experimental group, the evaluators will be on firmer ground in concluding that the program is effective (Example 3.2).

Example 3.2 An Effective Literacy Program: Hypothetical Example

Assignment	Before the Program	After the Program
Randomly assigned to the experimental literacy program	Relatively weak writing skills	Significantly improved writing skills
Randomly assigned to a comparable literacy program	Relatively weak writing skills	No change: Writing skills are still relatively weak

Conclusion: The experimental program effectively improved writing skills when compared to a comparable program.

In sum, randomized controlled trials are controlled experiments where evaluators compare two or more programs, interventions, or practices in eligible individuals or groups who receive them in random order.

Two commonly used randomized control designs are:

- **Parallel controls** in which two (or more) groups are randomly constituted, and they are studied at the same time (parallel to one another); and
- **Waitlist controls** where one group receives the program first and others are put on a waiting list; then if the program appears to be effective, participants on the waiting list receive it. Participants are randomly assigned to the experimental and waitlist groups.

Parallel Controls

An evaluation design using parallel controls is one where programs are compared to each other at the same time (in parallel). The design requires three steps:

1. The evaluators assess the eligibility of potential participants.
   - Some people are excluded because they do not satisfy the evaluation's inclusion criteria (must be a certain age; must have a particular medical condition) or they satisfy the exclusion criteria (refuse to give their email address; do not have reliable internet access).
   - Some eligible people decide not to participate. They change their mind, become ill, or are too busy.
2. The eligible and willing participants are enrolled in the evaluation study.
3. These same participants are randomly assigned to the experiment (one or more programs) or to an alternative (the control, which can be one or more comparison programs).

How does this work in practice? Suppose an evaluation is planned to compare the effectiveness of three programs for women whose partners are substance abusers. The three programs are:

1. Online partner substance abuse screening measure plus a list of local resources.
2. A list of local resources only.
3. Usual treatment program or another program which is left to the women to select on their own.

Evidence of effectiveness is a significant difference in quality of life among the three groups over a one-year period. The evaluators anticipate that the difference will be in favor of the new and most intensive intervention: computerized partner substance abuse screen and resource list.

Women are eligible for the evaluation if they are at least 18 years of age and have a working phone. Women are excluded from participation if they are accompanied by their partner during the selection process and cannot be safely separated at the enrollment site.

Figure 3.1 shows how the design for this study played out over the course of the evaluation. As you see from the figure, of the 3,537 women who were contacted originally, 2,708 or 76% were eligible for randomization. About 87% of the 2,708 completed the one-year follow-up.

The figure shows the flow of three groups of participants through a randomized controlled trial of a program for people whose partners have substance abuse problems. The figure starts by showing the number of people who are approached to participate (n = 3,537) and continues with the number who were considered eligible (2,708) and subsequently randomized to two experimental groups and one control. The figure then shows the number of people who were lost to follow-up (386). The figure's flow concludes with the number of people in each of the three study groups who completed the evaluation after one year (Experimental group 1, screen plus resources = 919, Experimental group 2, resources only = 843, and Usual Care = 938).

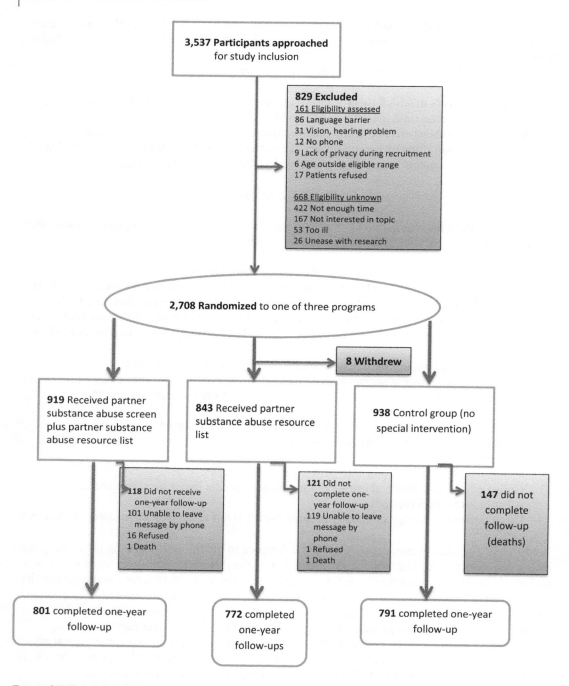

Figure 3.1 Randomized Controlled Trial Flow: From Inclusion to Completion

Waitlist Controls

With a waitlist control design, both groups are measured for eligibility, but one is randomly assigned to be given the program now—the experimental group— and the other—the control— is put on a waiting list. After the experimental group completes the program, both groups are measured a second time. Then the control receives the program and both groups are measured again (Figure 3.2)

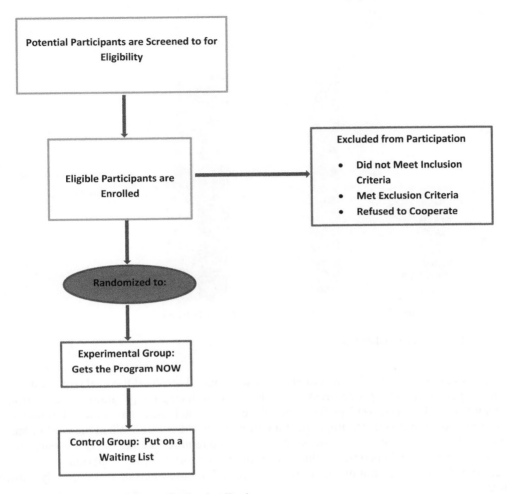

Figure 3.2 Waitlist Control Group Evaluation Design

The figure depicts a waitlist control design flow. The flow includes assessing participants for eligibility, then enrolling them. After enrollment, the figure shows that participants are randomized to an experimental group that receives the program immediately, while the controls are put on a waitlist to receive the program after the experimental group is finished with its participation.

Here is how the waitlist design is used:

1. Compare Group 1 (experimental group) and Group 2 (control group) at baseline (the pretest). If random assignment has "worked," the two groups should not differ from one another.
2. Give Group 1—the experimental group—the program.
3. Assess the outcomes for Groups 1 and 2 at the end of the program. If the program is effective, expect to see a difference in outcomes favoring the experimental group.
4. Give the program to Group 2.
5. Assess the outcomes a second time. If the program is effective, Group 2 should catch up to Group 1, and both should have improved in their outcomes (Figure 3.3).

Waitlist control designs are practical when programs are repeated at regular intervals, as they are in schools with a semester system. Students, for example, can be randomly assigned to Group 1 or Group 2, with Group 1 participating in the first semester. Group 2 can then participate in the second semester.

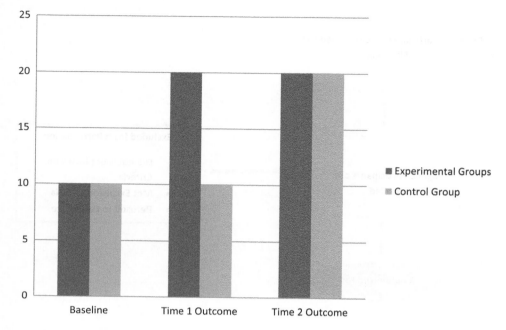

Figure 3.3 The Waitlist Catches Up

Waitlist control designs are most likely to yield unbiased results if the evaluator waits until the experimental group's progress ceases before introducing the program to the control. This wait is called a "wash-out" period. Once the experimental group has achieved as much as it is going to, then it is fair to implement the program in the control. When the control has completed the program, another wash-out period may be required so that the two groups are compared at their "true" maximum achievement points. Unfortunately, the amount of time needed for effects to wash out in either the experimental or control group is not usually known in advance.

RANDOMIZING AND BLINDING

Random Assignment

Randomization is the primary method of ensuring that participant groups are alike at baseline—that is, before they participate in a program. The idea behind randomization is that if chance—which is what random means—dictates the allocation to programs, all important factors will be equally distributed between the experimental and the control group. No single factor will dominate any of the groups, possibly influencing program outcomes. That is, to begin with, each group will be as smart, as motivated, as knowledgeable, and as self-efficacious as the other. As a result, any differences between or among groups that are observed later, after program participation, can reasonably be assigned to the program rather than to the differences that were there at the beginning. In evaluation terms, randomized controlled trials result in unbiased estimates of a program's effects.

How does random assignment work? Consider the following commonly used method (Example 3.3).

Example 3.3 Random Assignment

1. An algorithm or set of rules is applied to a table of random numbers, which are usually generated by computer. For instance, if the evaluation design includes an experimental and a control group and an equal probability of being assigned to each, then the algorithm could specify using the random number 1 for assignment to the experimental group and 2 for assignment to the control group.
2. As each eligible person enters the study, he or she is assigned one of the numbers (1 or 2).
3. The random assignment procedure should be designed so that members of the evaluation team who have contact with participants cannot influence the allocation process. For instance, random assignments to experimental or control groups can be placed in advance in a set of sealed envelopes by someone who will not be involved in their distribution. Each envelope can be numbered so that all can be accounted for by the end of the evaluation. As a participant comes through the system, his or her name is recorded, the envelope is opened, and then the assignment (1 or 2) is recorded next to the person's name.
4. It is crucial in randomized controlled trials that the evaluators prevent interference with randomization. Who would tamper with assignment? Sometimes, members of the evaluation team may feel pressure to ensure that the neediest people receive the experimental program. One method of avoiding this is to ensure that tamper-proof procedures are in place. If the research team uses envelopes, they should ensure the envelopes are opaque (so no one can see through them) and sealed. In large studies, randomization is typically done away from the site.

Random Clusters

Some evaluations randomly assign *clusters* of individuals (such as families or communities) rather than individuals to the experimental or control groups. Suppose an evaluation aims to study the effectiveness of a college-based smokeless tobacco cessation program for college athletes. The evaluators define effectiveness as reported cessation of smokeless tobacco use in the previous 30 days.

Current users of smokeless tobacco (defined as those who use more than once per month and within the past month) are eligible for the evaluation. The evaluators select 16 colleges with an average of 23 smokeless tobacco users, and randomly assign eight colleges to an experimental program and eight to a control. Both the experimental and control groups are asked about their smokeless tobacco use before the evaluation begins and three months after its conclusion. The evaluators then compare the experimental and control groups to find out if differences existed in tobacco use in the previous 30 days.

Please note that in this example, data on the outcome (cessation of smokeless tobacco use in the previous 30 days) was collected from individual students, but randomization was done by college—not by student. Is this OK? The answer depends on how the evaluation deals with the potential problems caused by randomizing with one unit (colleges) and analyzing data from another (students).

Here are seven questions to answer when reporting on a cluster randomized trial. The answers to these questions have implications for analyzing the data and coming to conclusions about whether the evaluation's conclusions apply to the cluster or to the individual.

Questions about clusters:

1. Do the evaluation questions refer to the cluster level, the individual participant level or both?
2. Do the programs pertain to the cluster level, the individual participant level, or both?
3. Do the outcome measures pertain to the cluster level, the participant level, or both?
4. How were people assigned to programs: by cluster or by participant?

5. How were individuals chosen for participation within each cluster? For example, were all classrooms within the experimental cluster of schools chosen? A sample? Were students sampled in some classrooms so that within any single classroom, some students were in the experimental group but others were in control?
6. How were participants informed about the evaluation? By cluster? Individually?
7. How do the clusters and individuals in the experimental and control group each compare at baseline? At follow-up? That is, did people differ in drop-out rates by group, cluster, and individual?

Improving on Chance: Stratifying and Blocking

Despite all efforts to do the right thing, chance may dictate that experimental and control groups differ on important variables at baseline even though they were randomized.

RCTs can gain power to detect a difference between experimental and control programs (assuming one is present) if special randomization procedures are used to balance the numbers of participants in each (*blocked randomization*) and in the distribution of baseline variables that might influence the outcomes (*stratified blocked randomization*).

Why are special procedures necessary if random assignment is supposed to take care of the number of people in each group or the proportion of people in each with certain characteristics?

The answer is that, by chance, one group may end up being larger than the other (differences in drop-out rate) or inherently different from the other with an unequal distribution of variables such as age (70% of the sample is between 20 and 30 years of age), gender (62% of the sample is male), and so on. Good news: This happens less frequently in large studies with carefully thought-out sampling plans. Bad news: The problem of unequal distribution of variables becomes even more complicated when clusters of people (schools or families) rather than individuals are assigned to programs.

Evaluators who use cluster assignment have no control over the individuals within each cluster, and the number of clusters over which they do have control is usually relatively small (e.g., five schools or ten clinics). Accordingly, some form of intervention, such as stratification, is almost always recommended in RCTs in which allocation is done by cluster.

Suppose a team of evaluators wants to be certain that the number of participants in each group is balanced. The team could use *blocks* of predetermined sizes. For example, if the block's size is six, the team will randomly assign three people to one group and three to the other group until the block of six is completed. This means that in an evaluation with 30 participants, 15 will be assigned to each group, and in a study of 33, the disproportion can be no greater than a ratio of 18:15.

Now, suppose the team wants to be certain that important independent or predictor variables are balanced between the experimental and control group. That is, the team wants to be sure that each group is equally healthy and motivated to stay in the study. The team can use a technique called stratification. Stratification means dividing participants into segments.

Participants can be divided into differing age groups (the stratum), or gender, or educational level. For instance, in a study of a community program to improve knowledge of how to prevent infectious disease, including colds and flu, having access to reliable transportation to attend education classes is a strong predictor of outcome. When evaluating such a program, it is probably a good idea to have similar numbers of people who have transportation (determined at baseline) assigned to each group. This can be done by dividing the study sample at baseline into participants with or without transportation (stratification by access to transportation), and then carrying out a blocked randomization procedure with each of these two strata.

Blinding

In some randomized studies, the participants and the evaluators do not know which participants are in the experimental or the control groups. This is called a *double-blind* experiment. When participants do not know, but evaluators do know which participants are in the experimental or the control groups, this is called a *blinded* trial. Participants, people responsible for program implementation or assessing program outcomes, and statistical analysts are all candidates for being blinded in a study.

Design experts maintain that blinding is as important as randomization in ensuring unbiased study results. Randomization, they say, eliminates confounding variables before the program is implemented—at baseline—but it cannot do away with *confounding* variables that occur as the study progresses.

A confounding variable is an extraneous variable in a statistical or research model that affects the dependent variables (outcomes) and was not originally considered or not accounted for statistically. Age, educational level, and motivation are sample baseline variables that can confound program outcomes. Confounding during a study can occur if experimental participants get extra attention, or the control group catches on to the experiment.

Confounders can lead to a false conclusion that the dependent variables are in a causal relationship with the independent or predictor variables. For instance, suppose research shows that drinking coffee (independent or predictor variable) is associated with heart attacks (the dependent variable). One possibility is that drinking coffee causes heart attacks. Another is that having heart attacks causes people to drink more coffee. A third explanation is that some other confounding factor, such as smoking, is responsible for heart attacks and is also associated with drinking coffee.

RCTs are generally expensive, requiring large teams of skilled evaluators. They tend to be disruptive in ordinary or real-world settings, and they are designed to answer very specific research questions. However, when implemented skillfully, they can provide strong evidence that Program A, when compared to Program B, causes participants with selected characteristics in selected settings to achieve selected benefits that last a given time.

NONRANDOMIZED CONTROLLED TRIALS

Parallel Controls

Nonrandomized controlled trials (sometimes called *quasi-experiments*) are designs in which one group receives the program and one does not, the assignment of participants to groups is not controlled by evaluators, and assignment is not random.

Nonrandomized controlled trials rely on participants who (1) volunteer to join the study, (2) are geographically close to the study site, or (3) conveniently turn up (at a clinic or school) while the study is being conducted. As a result, people or groups in a nonrandomized trial may self-select, and the evaluation findings may be biased because they are dependent on participant choice rather than chance.

Nonrandomized trials rely on a variety of methods to ensure that the participating groups are as like one another as possible (equivalent) at baseline or before intervention. Among the strategies used to ensure equivalence is *matching*.

Matching means selecting pairs of participants who are comparable to one another on important confounding variables, such as age or motivation, and then randomly assigning them to either the experimental or control group.

Matching is often problematic. For one thing, it is sometimes difficult to identify the variables to match, and even if you do identify them, you may not have access to reliable measures of these variables (such as a measure of motivation to learn, or a measure of patient safety) or the time and resources to administer them. Also, for each variable that you measure, another equally important variable (experience, knowledge, health) may not be measured. Evaluators who use matching typically use statistical techniques to "correct" for baseline differences and account for the many variables that matching excludes.

Other methods for allocating participants to study groups in nonrandomized evaluations include assigning each potential participant a number and using an alternating sequence in which every other individual (1, 3, 5, etc.) is assigned to the experimental group and the alternate participants (2, 4, 6, etc.) are assigned to the control. Another option is to assign groups in order of appearance so, for example, patients who attend the clinic on Monday, Wednesday, and Friday are in the experimental group, and those attending on Tuesday, Thursday, and Saturday are assigned to the control.

Strong nonrandomized designs have many desirable features. They can provide information about programs when it is inappropriate or too late to randomize participants. Also, when compared to RCTs, nonrandomized trials tend to fit more easily into and accurately reflect how a program is likely to function in the real world. RCTs require strict control over the environment, and to get that control, the evaluator must be extremely stringent with respect to selection and exclusion of study participants. As a result, RCT findings generally apply to a relatively small population in constrained settings.

Well-designed nonrandomized trials are difficult to plan and implement and require the highest level of evaluation expertise. Many borrow techniques from RCTs, including blinding. Many others use sophisticated statistical methods to enhance confidence in the findings.

The Problem of Incomparable Participants: Statistical Methods like ANCOVA to the Rescue

In nonrandomized studies, the evaluator cannot assume that the experimental and control groups are alike before participation. But if the participants are different to begin with, how can the evaluator who finds a difference between experimental and control outcomes separate the effects of the intervention from differences in study participants? One answer is to consider taking care of potential confounders (education, motivation to succeed) during the data analysis phase by using statistical methods like analysis of covariance or ANCOVA.

A confounding variable, also known as a *mediator variable* or *covariate*, is related to the independent variable and can adversely affect the relationship between the independent and outcome variables. A researcher who studies the cause of heart attacks, for example, will probably consider age as a probable confounding variable because heart attacks occur more frequently in older people. Analysis of covariance (ANCOVA) is a statistical procedure that can be used to adjust for confounding variables.

Suppose an evaluation is interested in assessing how effective an experimental tenth-grade mathematics program is in improving algebra skills as compared to the traditional program. Several confounding variables such as age or motivation can affect the assessment unless a method can be found to neutralize them. ANCOVA is a statistical method that can be used so that the confounding variables are neutralized or controlled.

When using ANCOVA, the evaluator of the tenth-grade mathematics program evaluation will "regress" the algebra skills of tenth graders on each confounding variable. Regression is a way of mathematically sorting out which of those variables has an impact on the dependent variables or outcomes (algebra skills). The regression will remove the variance in algebra skills that is due to the confounding variables or covariates (age and motivation), leaving only the variance that is due to the mathematics program. The program can then be tested for its effects on algebra skills. If the results of the ANCOVA show that students in the experimental program have significantly greater algebra skills at the program's conclusion, the evaluator can conclude that the experimental program is comparatively effective in achieving its goal.

Which covariates are potentially linked to outcomes? To find out, the evaluator reviews the literature, gathers expert opinion, or conducts research studies. The evaluators must justify their choice of covariates by providing evidence that age or motivation is related to learning algebra skills.

ANCOVA is one among several statistical methods for controlling confounding variables. Among them are sensitivity analysis, instrumental variables analysis, and propensity score analysis. Each of these makes assumptions about the nature and distribution of the data that is collected to measure the independent, dependent or outcome, and confounding variables. Statistical expertise is essential in selecting and implementing the appropriate strategy to control potential confounders.

OBSERVATIONAL EVALUATION DESIGNS

When evaluators use *observational designs*, they describe events (cross-sectional or survey designs), or examine them as they occur (cohort designs), or describe events that have already taken place (case control designs).

Cross-Sectional Designs

Evaluators use cross-sectional designs to collect baseline information on experimental and control groups, to guide program development, and to survey people to get their opinion. The data used in these designs come from questionnaires, reviews of documents and records, achievement tests, observations, and interviews. Cross-sectional designs enable evaluators to develop portraits of one or many groups at one time. Example 3.4 illustrates three uses of cross-sectional designs.

Example 3.4 Cross-Sectional or Survey Designs and Program Evaluation

1. *Randomly ordered and anonymous physician and chatbot responses*: Evaluators used a public and nonidentifiable database of questions from a public social media forum to randomly draw 195 exchanges in which a verified physician responded to a public question. Chatbot responses were generated by entering the original question into a fresh session. A team of health care professionals reviewed all responses. They chose "which response was better," and judged "the quality of information provided" (*very poor, poor, acceptable, good*, or *very good*) and "the empathy or bedside manner provided" (*not empathetic, slightly empathetic, moderately empathetic, empathetic*, and *very empathetic*).

Average (mean) outcomes were ordered on a 1 to 5 scale and compared between chatbot and physicians. Of the 195 questions and responses, reviewers preferred chatbot responses to physician responses in 78.6% (95% CI, 75.0%–81.8%) of the 585 reviews. The evaluators concluded that in this cross-sectional study, a chatbot generated quality and empathetic responses to patient questions posed in an online forum. They recommended that additional exploration of this technology is warranted in clinical settings, such as using chatbot to draft responses that physicians could then edit.

Comment: A cross-sectional survey of chatbot and physician responses reviewed to determine if AI technology is warranted in clinical settings.

2. *A test of student knowledge of program evaluation principles*: The Curriculum Committee wanted information on entering social work graduate students' knowledge of the methods and uses of program evaluation in improving social welfare. The committee asked the evaluator to prepare

and administer a brief test to all students. The results revealed that 80% could not distinguish between cross-sectional and experimental evaluation designs, and only 20% could list more than one source for setting standards of program merit. The Curriculum Committee used these findings to develop a course of instruction to provide entering graduate students with the skills they need to conduct and review evaluations.

Comment: The test is used in a cross-sectional survey of students to get information on curriculum content.

3. *A review of the care of hypertensive patients:* Evaluators conducted a review of the medical records of 2,500 patients in three medical centers to find out about the management of patients with hypertension. They are using the data to determine whether a program is needed to improve dissemination of practice guidelines for this common medical problem and to determine how that program should be evaluated.

Comment: The cross-sectional review or survey of medical records is used to guide program development.

Cohort Designs

A *cohort* is a group of people who share a common problem or characteristic (e.g., smoking during pregnancy) and who remain part of a study over an extended period. Consider, for example, a team of evaluators which is interested in investigating whether a new program to educate pregnant women about the potentially harmful effects of smoking on their children's IQ can be justified. To begin the investigation, the evaluators identify the cohort—in this instance, pregnant women who smoke. Then, they follow the women *prospectively* for a given time period, say five years. (Example 3.5).

Example 3.5 A Cohort Design

The evaluation team was interested in finding out if there is a need for a program to educate pregnant women about the potentially harmful effects of smoking on their children's IQ. They conducted a prospective follow-up study on a cohort of 1,782 women and their offspring who were sampled from the National Birth Cohort Registry. Five years later, the children were tested with the Wechsler Preschool and Primary Scale of Intelligence-Revised (WPPSI-R). The evaluator compared the IQ of children whose mothers smoked with the IQ of children whose mothers did not smoke.

In this prospective observational study, the evaluator did not introduce a program. The study was instead performed to investigate whether there is a need for a program. High-quality prospective or *longitudinal* studies are expensive to conduct, especially if the evaluator is concerned with outcomes that are hard to predict, as is IQ (Example 3.5). Studying unpredictable outcomes requires large samples and numerous measures.

Evaluators who do prospective cohort studies have to be on guard against loss of subjects over time or *attrition.* Longitudinal studies of children, for example, are characterized by attrition because, over time, families lose interest, move far away, change their names, and so on. If many people drop out of a study or cannot be found, the sample that remains may be very different from the initial one in such factors as age, motivation, or health.

Case Control Designs

Case control studies compare people who have a particular condition (the cases) to people who do not have the condition (the controls). The researchers look back in time to try to identify the factors that are unique to the cases and may have contributed to the development of the condition. For example, in a study that hypothesizes that people who smoke are more likely to be diagnosed with lung cancer, the *cases* are people with lung cancer, and the *controls* are people without lung cancer. To find out if smoking differentiates the cases from the control, the researchers analyze an existing database—that is, they go back in time through the data. If they find that the cases differ from the controls because a significantly larger number of them smoke, then their hypothesis is supported. The researchers can say that smoking came before lung cancer. Case controls are *retrospective* or historical studies.

Case control studies cannot prove that one thing causes another. They can only show that there is an association between two things. For example, in the study of smoking and lung cancer, it is possible that there are some other factors causing both the smoking and the cancer. Nevertheless, despite their inability to establish causation, case control studies can be a valuable tool for evaluators because they can provide clues to the characteristics of people who may benefit most from a planned or existing program. And because these designs use existing databases, the information they provide can be based on very large numbers of people at a relatively low cost. They are limited, however, to whatever information is contained in the database.

A Note on Pretest-Posttest Only or Self-Controlled Designs

In a simple pretest-posttest only design (also called self-controlled design), participants are measured on some important program variable (e.g., quality of life) and serve as their own control. These designs do not have a separate control group. Participants are usually measured twice (at baseline and after program participation), but they may be measured multiple times before and after as well. For instance, the evaluators of a new one-year program decided to collect data five weeks before participation, at enrollment, and at intervals of three, six, and 12 months after program completion. The data was subsequently used to modify the program based on participant feedback. At the conclusion of the 12-month period, the evaluators felt confident that the program was ready for implementation.

Pretest-posttest designs are not appropriate for effectiveness evaluations. They tend to be relatively small and limited in duration, and because they have no control group, they are subject to many potential biases. For instance, between the pretest and the posttest, participants may mature physically, emotionally, and intellectually, thereby affecting the program's outcomes. Without a comparison, you cannot tell if any observed changes are due to the new program or to maturation. Finally, self-controlled evaluations may be affected by historical events, including changes in program administration and policy. You need a comparison group that is also subject to the same historical events to understand the likely reason for any change you observe: Is the change due to the program or the event?

FACTORIAL DESIGNS

Factorial designs enable evaluators to measure the effects of varying the features of a program or practice to see which combination works best. In Example 3.6, the evaluators are concerned with finding out if the response rate to web-based surveys can be improved by notifying prospective responders in advance by email and/or pleading with them to respond. The evaluators design a study to solve the response-rate problem using a two-by-two (2 X 2) factorial design where participants are either notified about the survey in advance by email or not notified in advance, or they are pleaded with to respond or not pleaded with.

The *factors* (they are also independent variables) are Pleading (Factor 1) and Notifying (Factor 2). Each factor has two "levels": Plead versus Don't Plead and Notify in Advance versus Don't Notify in Advance.

Example 3.6 Factorial Design

Factor 2: Notification Status	Factor 1: Pleading Status	
	Plead	**Don't Plead**
Notify in Advance		
Don't Notify in Advance		

In a two-by-two or 2 X (times) 2 factorial design, there are four study groups: (1) advance notification email and pleading invitation email; (2) advance notification email and non-pleading invitation; (3) no advance notification email and pleading invitation; (4) no advance notification and non-pleading invitation. In the example above, the empty cells are placeholders for the number of people in each category, such as the number of people in the groups under the categories "Plead" and "Notify in Advance" compared to the number of people under "Plead" and "Don't Notify in Advance."

With this design, evaluators can study *main effects* (plead versus don't plead) or *interactive effects* (advance notification and pleading). The outcome in this study is the response rate.

Factorial designs can include many factors and many levels. It is the number of levels that describes the type of design. For instance, in a study of psychotherapy versus behavior modification in outpatient, inpatient, and day treatment settings, there are two factors (treatment and setting), with one factor having two levels (psychotherapy versus behavior modification) and one factor having three levels (inpatient, day treatment, and outpatient). This design is a 2 X 3 factorial design.

The study is a randomized controlled trial if the selection of a group for the research participants is a random assignment.

NON-INFERIORITY EVALUATION DESIGNS

Non-inferiority evaluation designs are used when a standard program is available and effective, but it is difficult or costly to implement. The idea is that if a new program can be shown to be non-inferior to the standard one—that is, it is at least not worse—then it can be considered an effective alternative to the standard program especially if it is easier to use or less expensive.

Suppose, for example, a university has commissioned an evaluation to compare the effectiveness of a new educational program (Program A) to its standard educational program (Program B) to determine if it can improve students' Grade Point Average (GPA) The reason for considering the new program is that it is much less expensive than the standard one. The evaluators suggest they do a non-inferiority evaluation, and the university agrees. The expectation is that if students in the new program do not do worse than students in the standard program, then the university will consider adopting it.

Evaluators sometimes find it difficult to justify a non-inferiority design to stakeholders who tend to be suspicious of supporting the evaluation of a new program if an effective one already exists. Their expectation is that if resources are to be spent on a new program, it should be demonstrably better than the existing one and not just "not worse." Nevertheless, despite its limitations, non-inferiority evaluation designs have gained favor because of their cost-savings potential. For instance, they have been used successfully to evaluate whether mental health programs that use remote methods, such as telehealth and teleconferencing for treatment, are potential alternatives to expensive and sometimes inaccessible in-person care.

COMPARATIVE EFFECTIVENESS EVALUATIONS

Comparative effectiveness evaluation designs are used in the health sciences (public health, medicine, nursing), but they are appropriate for all disciplines (education, psychology, social work). These evaluations aim to compare the health outcomes and clinical effectiveness, risks, and benefits of two or more available health or medical treatments, programs, or services.

Comparative effectiveness evaluations or research (CER) have four defining characteristics:

1. Two programs are directly compared with one another. For instance, Program A to improve immunization rates is compared to Program B to improve immunization rates.
2. The standard of effectiveness is explicit. For example, Program A is effective when compared to Program B, if it achieves all its five stated objectives *and* costs less per participant than Program B.
3. The patients, clinicians, and programs who participate in the evaluation must be representative of usual practice. Programs A and B take place in naturalistic settings (doctors' offices, clinics, hospitals) and often involve already existing activities (reminders to patients to get immunized).
4. The goal of the evaluation is to help everyday patients, clinicians, and policy makers make informed choices by providing the best available evidence on the effectiveness, quality, and value of alternative programs.

One unique characteristic of comparative effectiveness evaluation or research (CER) is its emphasis on having study activities take place in usual practice rather than in controlled settings. In typical evaluations, the evaluators alter or control the environment. They may include only people with certain characteristics (e.g., people without chronic illness) and exclude others (e.g., people with high blood pressure or depression). In CER, all these people are eligible to be in the study because, in real life, the physician or hospital does not exclude them from care.

A second unique characteristic of CER is found in its primary purpose: to provide information for improved decision making. The questions CER practitioners ask when designing their studies are: Will the findings provide a patient, clinician, or policymaker with information to make a more informed choice than they would have without the evaluation? Did the evaluation promote informed decision making? Example 3.7 summarizes two comparative effectiveness evaluations.

Example 3.7 Comparative Effectiveness Evaluations in Action

1. Are helicopter or ground emergency medical services more effective for adults who have suffered a major trauma? (Galvagno et al., 2012)

Helicopter services are a limited and expensive resource, and their effectiveness is subject to debate. The evaluators compared the effectiveness of helicopter and ground emergency services in caring for trauma patients. They defined one standard of effectiveness as survival to hospital discharge. Data was collected from the American College of Surgeons National Trauma Data Bank on 223,475 patients older than 15 years, having an injury severity score considered "high," and sustaining blunt or penetrating trauma that required transport to U.S. Level I or Level II trauma centers.

The study found that a total of 61,909 patients were transported by helicopter, and 161,566 patients were transported by ground. Overall, 7,813 patients (12.6%) transported by helicopter died compared with 17,775 patients (11%) transported by ground services. Helicopter transport, when compared with ground transport, was associated with improved odds of survival for patients transported to both Level I and Level II trauma centers. These findings were significant. Concurrently, fewer patients transported by helicopter left Level II trauma centers against medical advice. These findings were also significant.

After controlling for multiple known confounders, the evaluators concluded that among patients with major trauma admitted to Level I or Level II trauma centers, that transport by helicopter compared with ground services was associated with improved survival to hospital discharge.

2. Is face-to-face or over-the-telephone delivery of cognitive-behavioral therapy more effective and cost-effective for patients with common mental disorders? (Hammond et al., 2012)

The evaluators collected data over a two-year period on 39,227 adults who were in a program to improve access to psychological services. Patients received two or more sessions of cognitive-behavioral therapy (CBT). The over-the-telephone delivery program was hypothesized to be no worse in improving outcomes than the face-to-face intervention. This is called a "non-inferiority" effectiveness standard.

Patients usually completed questionnaires for depression, anxiety, and work and social adjustment, and the evaluators used these existing questionnaire data in the analysis. As hypothesized, they found that the over-the-telephone intervention was no worse than the face-to-face intervention, except in the case of the most ill patients. The telephone intervention, however, cost 36.3% less than the face-to-face intervention. The evaluators concluded that, given the non-inferiority of the telephone intervention, the evaluation provided evidence for better targeting of psychological therapies for people with common mental disorders.

The first illustration in Example 3.7 is a comparative effectiveness evaluation because:

1. Two programs (helicopter and ground emergencies) are compared to one another.
2. The standard of effectiveness is explicit: survival to hospital discharge.
3. The evaluators use data taken from actual emergency events. They do not create a special environment to observe what happens to trauma patients.

AND

4. The evaluators provide information on which of the two interventions is more effective to help inform choices between the two.

The second illustration is a comparative effectiveness evaluation because:

1. Two programs are compared: face-to-face versus over-the-telephone cognitive-behavioral therapy.
2. The standard is explicit: Over-the-telephone intervention will not be inferior to face-to-face ("non-inferiority").
3. The evaluators use data that was collected as a routine part of treatment; they do not collect new data.

AND

4. The evaluators provide data on effectiveness and cost-effectiveness to better inform decisions about which intervention to choose.

CER or pragmatic evaluations are costly and tend to involve large numbers of people in many settings, requiring teamwork, and statistical expertise.

COMMONLY USED EVALUATION DESIGNS

Program evaluators in the real world must make trade-offs when designing a study. Table 3.1 describes the benefits and concerns of eight basic evaluation designs.

Table 3.1 Eight Basic Program Evaluation Designs: Benefits and Concerns

Evaluation Design	Benefits	Concerns
Design with parallel controls and random assignment (randomized controlled trial; true experiment)	Can establish the extent to which a program caused outcomes.	Difficult to implement logistically and methodologically. Answers very specific research questions. May not reflect the real world because of stringent eligibility requirements and the logistics of randomization.
Design with parallel controls without randomization (quasi-experiment)	May be easier to implement than a randomized controlled trial.	May result in a wide range of potential biases because without equal chances of selection, participants in the program may be systematically different from those in the control group.
Cross-sectional design	Used to provide data on participant characteristics.	Offers a static picture of participants and program at one or more points in time.
Cohort design	Provides longitudinal or follow-up information.	Can be expensive because of the evaluation's long-term nature. Evaluators may have little say regarding which data is collected and how often. Participants who remain over time may differ in important ways from those who do not. Historical events can influence large groups of people.
Case control design	Can provide data on very large samples of people. No new data collection is needed. Can test the hypothesis that A may have caused B, with A occurring before B.	Relies on data that was collected previously for other purposes, and so the data may not be entirely appropriate for the current evaluation. Cannot establish causation.
Factorial design	Expands the possible number of evaluation questions possible and therefore the number of variables studied. Allows the study of main effects and interaction effects.	May need large numbers of people to collect valid data if there are large numbers of variables. May obtain false results if many statistical tests are performed to help answer a long list of questions.
Non-inferiority design	Provides information on new programs that are easier to implement, less costly, and "not worse" than the standard ones.	Sometimes it is difficult to justify their use because the standard program is already effective, and new programs and evaluations are expensive. The expectation is that if resources are to be spent on a new program it should be better, not just "not worse."
Comparative effectiveness evaluations	Provides information about program effectiveness, quality, and value in usual practice. Contributes to informed decision making by providing data on how programs perform with respect to specific standards of effectiveness, quality, and value.	These studies can be costly, requiring large numbers of people and a staff that is trained to do research and evaluation.

INTERNAL AND EXTERNAL VALIDITY

Internal validity refers to the extent to which the design and conduct of an evaluation are likely to have prevented bias. A study has internal validity if you report that Program A causes outcome A, and you can prove it with valid—that is, unbiased—evidence. An evaluation study has *external validity* if its results are applicable—*generalizable*—to other programs, populations, and settings. A study has external validity when, if you report that Program A can be used in Setting B, you can prove it with valid evidence.

Internal Validity Is Threatened

Just as the best laid plans of mice and men and women often go awry, evaluations, regardless of how well they are planned, lose something in their implementation. Randomization may not produce equivalent study groups, for example, or people in one study group may drop out more often than people in the other. Factors such as less than perfect randomization and attrition can threaten or bias an evaluation's findings. There are at least nine common threats to internal validity:

1. **Selection of participants:** This threat occurs when program groups are not equivalent at baseline. Perhaps the random assignment did not work or attempts to match groups or control for baseline confounders were ineffective. If participants are inherently different to begin with, the effects of these differences on the program's outcomes will be difficult to explain, trace, and measure. Selection can interact with history, maturation, and instrumentation.

2. **History:** Unanticipated events can occur while the evaluation is in progress, and this history will jeopardize internal validity. For instance, the effects of a school-based program to encourage healthier eating may be affected by a healthy eating campaign on a popular children's television show or social media.

3. **Maturation:** Program participants may grow physically and emotionally over time, threatening internal validity. Children in a three-year school-based physical education program mature physically, for example.

4. **Testing:** This threat can occur because taking one test influences the scores of a subsequent test. For instance, before and after a three-week program, participants are given a test. They recall their answers on the first test, and this influences their responses to the second test. The influence may be positive (they learn from the test) or negative (they recall incorrect answers).

5. **Instrumentation:** Changes in a measuring instrument or changes in observers or scorers cause an effect that can bias the results. Evaluator A makes changes to the questions in a structured interview given to participants at Time 1; she administers the changed questions in Time 2. Or, no changes are made in interview questions, but Evaluator A is replaced by Evaluator B; each evaluator has differing interview styles.

6. **Statistical regression:** Regression occurs when participants are selected based on extreme scores (very ill or in great need of assistance), and then, with time, they regress or go back toward an average score. Regression to the mean is a statistical artifact: its occurrence is due to some factor or factors outside of the evaluation.

7. **Attrition (drop-out) or loss to follow-up:** This threat to internal validity refers to the differential loss of participants from one or more groups on a nonrandom basis. Participants in one group drop out more frequently than participants in the others, or more are lost to follow-up, for example. The resulting two groups, which were alike to begin with, now probably differ.

8. **Expectancy:** A bias is caused by the expectations of the evaluator or the participants or both. Participants in the experimental group expect special treatment, while the evaluator expects to give it to them (and sometimes does). Blinding is one method of dealing with expectancy. A second is to ensure that a standardized process is used in delivering the program.

9. **Interruption:** An evaluation may be interrupted because of serious natural events such as fires, tsunamis, floods, epidemics, and pandemics. These interruptions can cause bias if substantial changes in staff occur when the evaluation resumes, and the new staff have different expectations of the evaluation. The evaluation's timeline may have to be shortened because of the interruption, forcing the evaluators to reduce the number of questions they can ask, recruit fewer or different participants, and collect fewer measurements.

External Validity Is Threatened

Threats to external validity are most often the consequence of the way in which participants or respondents are selected and assigned. They also occur whenever respondents are tested, surveyed, or observed. They may become alert to the kinds of behaviors that are expected or favored. There are at least four relatively common sources of external invalidity:

1. **Interaction effects of selection biases and the experimental treatment:** This threat to external validity occurs when a program and its participants are a unique mixture, one that may not be found elsewhere. The threat is most apparent when groups are not randomly constituted. Suppose a large company volunteers to participate in an experimental program to improve the quality of employees' leisure-time activities. The characteristics of the company, such as its leadership and priorities, are related to the fact that it volunteered for the experiment, and these characteristics may interact with the program so that the two elements combined make the study unique. Therefore, the blend of company and program can limit the applicability of the findings to other companies.

2. **Reactive effects of testing:** This threat occurs because participants are pretested, which sensitizes them to the treatment that follows. In fact, pretesting has such a powerful effect that teachers sometimes use pretests to get students ready for their next class assignment. A pretested group is different from one that has not been pretested, and so the results of an evaluation using a pretest may not be generalizable.

3. **Reactive effects of experimental arrangements or the Hawthorne effect:** This threat to external validity can occur when people know that they are participating in an experiment. Sometimes known as the *Hawthorne effect*, this threat is caused when people behave uncharacteristically because they are aware that their circumstances are different. They are being observed by cameras in the classroom, for instance.

4. **Multiple program interference:** This threat results when participants are in other complementary activities or programs that interact. Participants in an experimental mathematics program are also taking a physics class and both teach differential calculus; hence, the possible interference.

How do the threats to internal and external validity promote bias? Consider the Work and Stress Program, a yearlong program to help reduce on-the-job stress. Eligible people can enroll in one of two variations of their chosen program. To find out if participants are satisfied with the quality of the program, both groups complete an in-depth questionnaire at the end of the year, and the evaluator compares the results.

This is a nonrandomized controlled trial. Its internal validity is potentially marred by the fact that the participants in the groups may be different from one another from the start.

More stressed people may choose one program over the other, for example. Also, because of the initial differences, the attrition or loss to follow-up may be affected if the only people to continue with the program are the motivated ones. The failure to create randomly constituted groups will jeopardize the study's external validity by the interactive effects of selection.

SUMMARY AND TRANSITION TO THE NEXT CHAPTER ON SAMPLING IN PROGRAM EVALUATIONS

This chapter focused on ways to structure an evaluation to produce unbiased information of program effectiveness, quality, and value. The chapter also discusses the benefits and concerns associated with experimental and observational designs. Randomized controlled trials are recommended for evaluators who want to establish causation, but these designs are difficult to implement. Nonrandomized trials and observational designs are often used in evaluations, and, if rigorously implemented, can provide useful, high-quality data. Comparative effectiveness research aims to provide data for informed decision making by providing data on the effectiveness, quality, and value of alternative programs.

The next chapter discusses sampling—that is, what you need to do when you cannot obtain an entire eligible population for your evaluation. Among the issues discussed are how to obtain a random sample and how to select a large enough sample so that if program differences truly exist, you will find them.

EXERCISES: CHAPTER 3

Exercise 1

Read the following description of an evaluation of the effectiveness of a school-based intervention for reducing children's symptoms of PTSD and depression resulting from exposure to violence.

1. Name the design.
2. List the evaluation questions or hypotheses.
3. Identify the evidence of merit.
4. Describe the eligibility criteria.
5. Describe whether and how participants were assigned.
6. Discuss the timing and frequency of the measures.

Sixth-grade students at two large middle schools in Los Angeles who reported exposure to violence and had clinical levels of symptoms of PTSD were eligible for participation in the evaluation. Students were randomly assigned to a ten-session standardized cognitive-behavioral therapy (the Cognitive-Behavioral Intervention for Trauma in Schools) early intervention group (n = 61) or to a waitlist delayed intervention comparison group (n = 65) conducted by trained school mental health clinicians. Students were evaluated before the intervention and three months after the intervention on measures assessing child-reported symptoms of PTSD and depression, parent-reported psychosocial dysfunction, and teacher-reported classroom problems.

Exercise 2

Name the threats to internal and external validity in the following two study discussions.

1. The Role of Alcohol in Boating Deaths

Although many potentially confounding variables were considered, we were unable to adjust for other variables that might affect risk, such as the boater's swimming ability, the operator's boating skills and experience, use of personal flotation devices, water and weather conditions, and the condition and seaworthiness of the boat. Use of personal flotation devices was low among control subjects (about 6.7% of adults in control boats), but because such use was assessed only at the boat level and not for individuals, it was impossible to include it in our analyses. Finally, although we controlled for boating exposure with the random selection of control subjects, some groups may have been underrepresented.

2. Violence Prevention in the Emergency Department

The study design would not facilitate a blinding process that may provide more reliable results. The study was limited by those youth who were excluded, lost to follow-up, or had incomplete documents. Unfortunately, the study population has significant mobility and was commonly unavailable when the case managers attempted to interview them. The study was limited by the turnover of case managers.

Exercise 3

Describe the advantages and limitations of commonly used research designs, including:

- Randomized controlled trials with concurrent and waitlist control groups.
- Quasi-experimental or nonrandomized designs with concurrent control groups.
- Observational designs, including cohorts, case controls, and cross-sectional surveys.

REFERENCES AND SUGGESTED READINGS

Galvagno, S.M., Jr., Haut, E.R., Zafar, S.N., et al. (2012). Association between helicopter vs ground emergency medical services and survival for adults with major trauma. *JAMA: The Journal of the American Medical Association*, *307*(15): 1602–1610.

Hammond, G.C., Croudace, T.J., Radhakrishnan, M., Lafortune, L., Watson, A., McMillan-Shields, F., & Jones, P.B. (2012). Comparative effectiveness of cognitive therapies delivered face-to-face or over the telephone: An observational study using propensity methods. *PLoS One*, *7*(9).

Examples of Randomized Controlled Trials

Baird, S.J., Garfein, R.S., McIntosh, C.T., & Ozler, B. (2012). Effect of a cash transfer programme for schooling on prevalence of HIV and herpes simplex type 2 in Malawi: A cluster randomised trial. *Lancet*, *379*(9823): 1320–1329. https://doi.org/10.1016/S0140-6736(11)61709-1

Buller, M.K., Kane, I.L., Martin, R.C., Grese, A.J., Cutter, G.R., Saba, L.M., & Buller, D.B. (2008). Randomized trial evaluating computer-based sun safety education for children in elementary school. *Journal of Cancer Education*, *23*: 74–79.

Butler, R.W., Copeland, D.R., Fairclough, D.L., et al. (2008). A multicenter, randomized clinical trial of a cognitive remediation program for childhood survivors of a pediatric malignancy. *Journal of Consulting and Clinical Psychology*, *76*: 367–378.

Chung, Y. & Huang, H.H. (2021). Cognitive-based interventions break gender stereotypes in kindergarten children. *International Journal of Environmental Research and Public Health*, *8*(24): 13052.

Coulton, S., Stockdale, K., Marchand, C., et al. (2017). Pragmatic randomised controlled trial to evaluate the effectiveness and cost effectiveness of a multi-component intervention to reduce substance use and risk-taking behaviour in adolescents involved in the criminal justice system: A trial protocol (RISKIT-CJS). *BMC Public Health*, *17*(1): 246.

DuMont, K., Mitchell-Herzfeld, S., Greene, R., Lee, E., Lowenfels, A., Rodriguez, M., & Dorabawila, V. (2008). Healthy Families New York (HFNY) randomized trial: Effects on early child abuse and neglect. *Child Abuse & Neglect*, *32*: 295–315.

Fagan, J. (2008). Randomized study of a prebirth coparenting intervention with adolescent and young fathers. *Family Relations*, *57*: 309–323.

Ghetti, C.M., Gaden, T.S., Bieleninik, Ł., et al. (2023). Effect of music therapy on parent-infant bonding among infants born preterm: A randomized clinical trial. *JAMA Network Open*, *6*(5): e2315750.

Gillam, S.L., Vaughn, S., Roberts, G., et al. (2023). Improving oral and written narration and reading comprehension of children at-risk for language and literacy difficulties: Results of a randomized clinical trial. *Journal of Educational Psychology*, *15*),) : 99–117.

Hardy, L.L., King, L., Kelly, B., Farrell, L., & Howlett, S. (2010). Munch and Move: Evaluation of a preschool healthy eating and movement skill program. *The International Journal of Behavioral Nutrition and Physical Activity*, *7*: 80.

Johnson, J.E., Friedmann, P.D., Green, T.C., Harrington, M., & Taxman, F.S. (2011). Gender and treatment response in substance use treatment-mandated parolees. *Journal of Substance Abuse Treatment*, *40*(3): 313–321. doi:10.1016/j.jsat.2010.11.013

Marczinski, C.A. & Stamates, A.L. (2013). Artificial sweeteners versus regular mixers increase breath alcohol concentrations in male and female social drinkers. *Alcoholism, Clinical and Experimental Research*, *37*(4): 696–702.

Muela, A., Aliri, J., Presa, B., & Gorostiaga, A. (2020). Randomised controlled trial of a treatment adherence programme for prisoners with mental health problems in Spain. *Criminal Behaviour and Mental Health: CBMH*, *30*(1): 6–15.

Nance, D.C. (2012). Pains, joys, and secrets: Nurse-led group therapy for older adults with depression. *Issues in Mental Health Nursing*, *33*(2): 89–95. doi:10.3109/01612840.2011.624258

Ochandorena-Acha, M., Terradas-Monllor, M., Nunes Cabrera, T.F., Torrabias Rodas, M., & Grau, S. (2022). Effectiveness of virtual reality on functional mobility during treadmill training in children with cerebral palsy: A single-blind, two-arm parallel group randomised clinical trial (VirtWalkCP Project). *BMJ Open*, *2*(11): e061988.

Poduska, J.M., Kellam, S.G., Wang, W., Brown, C.H., Ialongo, N.S., & Toyinbo, P. (2008). Impact of the Good Behavior Game, a universal classroom-based behavior intervention, on young adult service use for problems with emotions, behavior, or drugs or alcohol. *Drug and Alcohol Dependence*, *95*: S29–S44.

Rdesinski, R.E., Melnick, A.L., Creach, E.D., Cozzens, J., & Carney, P.A. (2008). The costs of recruitment and retention of women from community-based programs into a randomized controlled contraceptive study. *Journal of Health Care for the Poor and Underserved*, *19*: 639–651.

Rosen, L., Zucker, D., Guttman, N., et al. (2021). Protecting children from tobacco smoke exposure: A randomized controlled trial of Project Zero Exposure. *Nicotine & Tobacco Research: Official Journal of the Society for Research on Nicotine and Tobacco*, *23*(12): 2003–2012.

Swart, L., van Niekerk, A., Seedat, M., & Jordaan, E. (2008). Paraprofessional home visitation program to prevent childhood unintentional injuries in low-income communities: A cluster randomized controlled trial. *Injury Prevention*, *14*(3): 164–169.

Thornton, J.D., Alejandro-Rodriguez, M., Leon, J.B., Albert, J.M., Baldeon, E.L., De Jesus, L.M., Sehgal, A.R. (2012). Effect of an iPod video intervention on consent to donate organs: A randomized trial. *Annals of Internal Medicine*, *156*(7): 483–490.

Vaezi, A. & Meysamie, A. (2021). COVID-19 vaccines cost-effectiveness analysis: A scenario for Iran. *Vaccines*, *10*(1): 37.

Examples of Nonrandomized Trials or Quasi-Experimental Studies

Chen, H., Zheng, X., Huang, H., Liu, C., Wan, Q., & Shang, S. (2020). The effects of a home-based exercise intervention on elderly patients with knee osteoarthritis: A quasi-experimental study. *BMC Musculoskeletal Disorders*, *20*(1): 160.

Corcoran, J. (2006). A comparison group study of solution-focused therapy versus "treatment-as-usual" for behavior problems in children. *Journal of Social Service Research*, *33*: 69–81.

Cross, T.P., Jones, L.M., Walsh, W.A., Simone, M., & Kolko, D. (2007). Child forensic interviewing in Children's Advocacy Centers: Empirical data on a practice model. *Child Abuse & Neglect*, *31*: 1031–1052.

Gatto, N.M., Ventura, E.E., Cook, L.T., Gyllenhammer, L.E., & Davis, J.N. (2012). L.A. Sprouts: A garden-based nutrition intervention pilot program influences motivation and preferences for fruits and vegetables in Latino youth. *Journal of the Academy of Nutrition and Dietetics*, *112*(6): 913–920. doi:10.1016/j.jand.2012.01.014

Hammond, G.C., Croudace, T.J., Radhakrishnan, M., et al. (2012). Comparative effectiveness of cognitive therapies delivered face-to-face or over the telephone: An observational study using propensity methods. *PloS One*, *7*(9): e42916.

Kutnick, P., Ota, C., & Berdondini, L. (2008). Improving the effects of group working in classrooms with young school-aged children: Facilitating attainment, interaction and classroom activity. *Learning and Instruction*, *18*: 83–95.

Lai, D.W.L., Ou, X., & Jin, J. (2022). A quasi-experimental study on the effect of an outdoor physical activity program on the well-being of older Chinese people in Hong Kong. *International Journal of Environmental Research and Public Health*. *19*(15): 35897322.

Marsh, T.N., Eshakakogan, C., Eibl, J.K., et al. (2021). A study protocol for a quasi-experimental community trial evaluating the integration of indigenous healing practices and a harm reduction approach with principles of seeking safety in an indigenous residential treatment program in Northern Ontario. *Harm Reduction Journal*, *18*(1): 35.

Stinson, C., Curl, E.D., Hale, G., et al. (2020). Mindfulness meditation and anxiety in nursing Students. *Nursing Education Perspectives*, *41*(4): 244–245.

Examples of Cohort Designs

Brown, C.S. & Lloyd, K. (2008). OPRISK: A structured checklist assessing security needs for men tally disordered offenders referred to high security psychiatric hospital. *Criminal Behaviour and Mental Health*, *18*: 190–202.

Chauhan, P. & Widom, C.S. (2012). Childhood maltreatment and illicit drug use in middle adult-hood: The role of neighborhood characteristics. *Development and Psychopathology*, *24*(3): 723–738. doi:10.1017/S0954579412000338

Dybvik, J.S., Svendsen, M., & Aune, D. (2023). Vegetarian and vegan diets and the risk of cardiovascular disease, ischemic heart disease and stroke: A systematic review and meta-analysis of prospective cohort studies. *European Journal of Nutrition, 62*(1): 51–69.

Galvagno, S.M., Jr., Haut, E.R., Zafar, S.N., et al. (2012). Association between helicopter vs ground emergency medical services and survival for adults with major trauma. *JAMA: The Journal of the American Medical Association, 307*(15): 1602–1610.

Kemp, P.A., Neale, J., & Robertson, M. (2006). Homelessness among problem drug users: Prevalence, risk factors and trigger events. *Health & Social Care in the Community, 14*: 319–328.

Kerr, T., Hogg, R.S., Yip, B., Tyndall, M.W., Montaner, J., & Wood, E. (2008). Validity of self-reported adherence among injection drug users. *Journal of the International Association of Physicians in AIDS Care, 7*(4): 157–159.

Nguyen, P.Y., Astell-Burt, T., Rahimi-Ardabili, H., & Feng, X. (2021). Green space quality and health: A systematic review. *International Journal of Environmental Research and Public Health, 8*(21): 11028.

Pletcher, M.J., Vittinghoff, E., Kalhan, R., et al. (2012). Association between marijuana exposure and pulmonary function over 20 years. *JAMA: The Journal of the American Medical Association, 307*(2): 173–181. doi:10.1001/jama.2011.1961

Van den Hooven, E.H., Pierik, F.H., de Kluizenaar, Y., et al. (2012). Air pollution exposure during pregnancy, ultrasound measures of fetal growth, and adverse birth outcomes: A prospective cohort study. *Environmental Health Perspectives, 120*(1): 150–156. doi:10.1289/ehp.1003316

Vieta, E. & Angst, J. (2021). Bipolar disorder cohort studies: Crucial, but underfunded. *European Neuropsychopharmacology: The Journal of the European College of Neuropsychopharmacology, 47*: 31–33.

White, H.R. & Widom, C.S. (2003). Does childhood victimization increase the risk of early death? A 25-year prospective study. *Child Abuse & Neglect, 27*: 841–853.

Examples of Case Control Studies

Belardinelli, C., Hatch, J.P., Olvera, R.L., et al. (2008). Family environment patterns in families with bipolar children. *Journal of Affective Disorders, 107*: 299–305.

Bookle, M. & Webber, M. (2011). Ethnicity and access to an inner city home treatment service: A case-control study. *Health & Social Care in the Community, 19*(3): 280–288.

Darabi, Z., Vasmehjani, A.A., Darand, M., Sangouni, A.A., & Hosseinzadeh, M. (2022). Adherence to Mediterranean diet and attention-deficit/hyperactivity disorder in children: A case control study. *Clinical Nutrition ESPEN, 47*: 346–350.

Davis, C., Levitan, R.D., Carter, J., et al. (2008). Personality and eating behaviors: A case-control study of binge eating disorder. *International Journal of Eating Disorders, 41*: 243–250.

Feda, D.M. (2012). Risk of physical assault against school educators with histories of occupational and other violence: A case-control study. *Work, 42*(1): 39–46.

Hall, S.S., Arron, K., Sloneem, J., & Oliver, C. (2008). Health and sleep problems in Cornelia de Lange syndrome: A case control study. *Journal of Intellectual Disability Research, 52*: 458–468.

Jiang, M., Mishu, M.M., Lu, D., & Yin, X. (2018). A case control study of risk factors and neonatal outcomes of preterm birth. (2018). *Taiwanese Journal of Obstetrics & Gynecology, 57*(6): 814–818.

Mohebbi, E., Rashidian, H., Naghibzadeh Tahami, A., et al. (2021). Opium use reporting error in case-control studies: Neighborhood controls versus hospital visitor controls. *Medical Journal of the Islamic Republic of Iran, 35*: 60.

Yu, J., He, H., Zhang, Y., et al. (2022). Burden of whooping cough in China (PertussisChina): Study protocol of a prospective, population-based case-control study. *BMJ Open, 12*(3): e053316.

Examples of Cross-Sectional Studies

Ayers, J.W., Poliak, A., Dredze, M., et al. (2023). Comparing physician and artificial intelligence chatbot Responses to patient questions posted to a public social media forum. *Journal of the American Medical Association Internal Medicine, 183*(6): 589–596.

Baminiwatta, A., Herath, N.C., & Chandradasa, M. (2021). Cross-sectional study on the association between social media use and body image dissatisfaction among adolescents. *Indian Journal of Pediatrics, 88*(5): 499–500.

Belardinelli, C., Hatch, J.P., Olvera, R.L., et al. (2008). Family environment patterns in families with bipolar children. *Journal of Affective Disorders*, *107*(1–3): 299–305.

Carmona, C.G.H., Barros, R.S., Tobar, J.R., Canobra, V.H., & Montequín, E.A. (2008). Family functioning of out-of-treatment cocaine base paste and cocaine hydrochloride users. *Addictive Behaviors*, *33*: 866–879.

Cooper, C., Robertson, M.M., & Livingston, G. (2003). Psychological morbidity and caregiver burden in parents of children with Tourette's disorder and psychiatric comorbidity. *Journal of the American Academy of Child & Adolescent Psychiatry*, *42*: 1370–1375.

Davis, C., Levitan, R.D., Carter, J., et al. (2008). Personality and eating behaviors: A case-control study of binge eating disorder. *International Journal of Eating Disorders*, *41*: 243–250.

DeBiasio, C., Li, H.O., Brandts-Longtin. O., & Kirchhof, M.G. (2022). Cannabis use in dermatology: A cross-sectional study of YouTube videos. *Journal of Cutaneous Medicine and Surgery*, *26*(6): 630–631.

Joice, S., Jones, M., & Johnston, M. (2012). Stress of caring and nurses' beliefs in the stroke rehabilitation environment: A cross-sectional study. *International Journal of Therapy & Rehabilitation*, *19*(4): 209–216.

Kypri, K., Bell, M.L., Hay, G.C., & Baxter, J. (2008). Alcohol outlet density and university student drinking: A national study. *Addiction*, *103*: 1131–1138.

Martinino, A., Scarano-Pereira, J.P., La Motta, E., et al. (2021). Healthy habits and Instagram: A cross-sectional study. *La Clinica Terapeutica*, *172*(3): 215–217.

Meijer, J.H., Dekker, N., Koeter, M.W., Quee, P.J., van Beveren, M.J.N., & Meijer, C.J. (2012). Cannabis and cognitive performance in psychosis: A cross-sectional study in patients with non-affective psychotic illness and their unaffected siblings. *Psychological Medicine*, *42*(4): 705–716. doi:10.1017/s0033291711001656

Schwarzer, R. & Hallum, S. (2008). Perceived teacher self-efficacy as a predictor of job stress and burnout. *Applied Psychology: An International Review*, *57*(Suppl. 1): 152–171.

ANSWERS TO THE EXERCISES: CHAPTER 3

Exercise 1

1. Experimental: randomized control trial or waitlist control.
2. **Hypothesis 1.** When compared to usual practice (delayed intervention), the Cognitive Behavioral Intervention for Trauma in Schools improves symptoms of PTSD and depression, parent-reported psychosocial dysfunction, and teacher-reported classroom problems at baseline (before the intervention) and three months later.
   Hypothesis 2. There will be no difference in symptoms, depression, dysfunction, and problems between students in the experimental and comparison programs three months after control students receive the experimental intervention.
3. Improvement in symptoms, depression, dysfunction, and problems for both the experimental and comparison group over a three-month period.
4. Sixth-grade students at two large middle schools in Los Angeles who reported exposure to violence and had clinical levels of symptoms of PTSD were eligible for participation in the evaluation.
5. No information is given on assignment.
6. Measures are administered twice: before the intervention and three months later.

Exercise 2

Answers are in bold and in parentheses except for commentary on this author's note concerning the second study.

The Role of Alcohol in Boating Deaths

Although many potentially confounding variables were taken into account, we were unable to adjust for other variables that might affect risk, such as the boater's swimming ability, the operator's boating skills and experience, use of personal flotation devices, water and weather conditions, and the condition and seaworthiness of the boat. Use of personal flotation devices was low among control subjects (about 6.7% of adults in control boats), but because such use was assessed only at the boat level and not for individuals, it was impossible to include it in our analyses (**Selection resulting in potentially nonequivalent groups**). Finally, although we controlled boating exposure with the random selections of control subjects, some groups may have been underrepresented (**Selection**).

Violence Prevention in the Emergency Department

The study design would not facilitate a blinding process (**Expectancy**) that may provide more reliable results. The study was limited by those youth who were excluded, lost to follow-up, or had incomplete documents (**Selection; Attrition**). Unfortunately, the study population has significant mobility and was commonly unavailable when the case managers attempted to interview them (**Attrition**). The study was limited by the turnover of case managers (**Attrition; Instrumentation**).

   Note: The first statement regarding the length of time needed for the program's effects to be observed is not a limitation in the study's research design, but in the evaluators' rush to try out a program with insufficient evidence. Limitations like this can be avoided in practice by relying only on programs that are known to work and that define the circumstances in which they work best.

   Regarding the second limitation concerning the evaluation tool, the problem here is that the evaluators used a measure of unknown validity. This is a serious (and not uncommon) problem. Invalid measures do harm to any study no matter how carefully it is designed. That is, a brilliantly designed RCT with an invalid test or other measure will produce inaccurate and biased results.

Exercise 3

RCTs with parallel and waitlist controls can guard against most biases. They produce the most internally and externally valid results. In their "purest" forms, however, they may be somewhat complex to implement. For example, it is often difficult, if not impossible, to "blind" all evaluation participants. Quasi-experimental designs are often more realistic for real-world environments like schools, prisons, and field settings. However, preexisting differences in groups may interfere with the results so that you cannot be certain if group differences or programs are responsible for outcomes.

Observational designs, like the case control design, make use of existing data. As a result, information can be collected on a very large sample for relatively little cost. However, the evaluators might not have had any say in how the original data was collected and from whom, and observational designs cannot establish causality.

Online or social media cross-sectional surveys can get responses from large samples at relatively low cost, but they only result in data that describes people at one point in time.

Cohort designs are subject to participant attrition and can take years to implement and complete.

CHAPTER 4 | SAMPLING IN PROGRAM EVALUATIONS

PURPOSE OF CHAPTER 4

Why do program evaluators typically use samples rather than entire populations of people in their studies? This chapter answers this question and discusses the advantages and limitations of five commonly used evaluation sampling methods: random, systematic, stratified, cluster, and convenience sampling. The chapter also explains the difference between unit of sampling (schools and hospitals) and the unit of data analysis (school or individual student, hospital, or individual patient) and discusses how to calculate an appropriate sample size. A form for reporting on sampling strategy is also offered. This form is designed to show the logical relationships among the evaluation questions, standards, independent variables, sampling strata, inclusion and exclusion criteria, dependent variables, measures, sampling methods, and sample size.

DOI: 10.4324/9781032635071-4

WHAT IS A SAMPLE?

A sample is a portion or subset of a larger group called a population. The evaluator's target population consists of the institutions, persons, problems, policies, and systems to which or to whom the evaluation's findings are to be applied or generalized. For example, suppose 500 students in one school who are 14 to 16 years of age are selected to be in an evaluation of a program to improve computer programming skills. If the program is effective, the school system's curriculum planners will offer it to all 14- to 16-year-olds throughout the system. The target population is students between the ages of 14 and 16. The school system may include thousands of 14- to 16-year-old students, but only a sample of 500 are included in the evaluation.

Consider the two target populations and samples in Example 4.1.

Example 4.1 Two Target Populations and Two Samples

Evaluation 1

Target population: All homeless military service veterans throughout the United States.
Program: Outreach, provision of single-room occupancy housing, medical and financial assistance, and job training: the REACH-OUT Program.
Sample: 500 homeless veterans in four of the fifty U.S. states who receive outpatient medical care between April 1 and June 30.

Evaluation 2

Target population: All newly diagnosed breast cancer patients.
Program: Education in Options for Treatment.
Sample: Five hospitals in three of the fifty U.S. states; within each hospital, 15 physicians; for each physician, 20 patients seen between January 1 and July 31 who are newly diagnosed with breast cancer.

The REACH-OUT Program in Evaluation 1 is designed for all homeless veterans. The evaluator plans to select a sample of 500 homeless veterans in four states between April 1 and June 30. The findings are to be applied to all homeless veterans in all 50 states. Women newly diagnosed with breast cancer are the targets of an educational program in Evaluation 2. The evaluators will select five hospitals, and, within them, 20 patients seen from January through July by each of 15 doctors. The findings are to be applied to all patients newly diagnosed with breast cancer.

WHY SAMPLE?

Evaluators sample because it is efficient, and because it contributes to the precision of their research. Samples can be studied more quickly than entire target populations, and they are also less expensive to assemble. In some cases, it would be impossible to recruit a complete population for an evaluation, even if the necessary time and financial resources were available. For example, it would be futile for an evaluator to attempt to enroll all prisoners or students or even a smaller population like homeless veterans in an investigation of a program that targets them (see Example 4.1).

Sampling is also efficient in that it allows the evaluator to invest resources in important evaluation activities, such as monitoring the quality of data collection and standardizing the implementation of the program, rather than in the collection of data on an unnecessarily large number of individuals or groups.

INCLUSION AND EXCLUSION CRITERIA OR ELIGIBILITY

A sample is a part of a larger population to which the evaluation's findings will be applied. If an evaluation is intended to investigate the impact of an educational program on women's knowledge of their options for surgical treatment for cancer, for example, and not all women with cancer are to be included in the program, the evaluator must decide on the characteristics of the women who will be the focus of the study. Will the evaluation concentrate on women of a specific age? Women with a particular kind of cancer? Example 4.2 presents hypothetical inclusion and exclusion criteria for an evaluation of such a program.

Example 4.2 Inclusion and Exclusion Criteria for a Sample of Women to Be Included in an Evaluation of a Program for Surgical Cancer Patients

Inclusion: Using the U.S. Medicare claims database, of all patients hospitalized during 2013, those with diagnosis or procedure codes related to breast cancer; for patients with multiple admissions, only the admission with the most invasive surgery.

Exclusion: Women under the age of 65 (because women under 65 who receive Medicare in the U.S. are generally disabled or have renal disease), men, women with only a diagnostic biopsy or no breast surgery, women undergoing bilateral mastectomy, women without a code for primary breast cancer at the time of the most invasive surgery, women with a diagnosis of carcinoma in situ, and women with metastases to regions other than the axillary lymph nodes.

The evaluator of this program has set criteria for the sample of women who will be included in the evaluation and for which its conclusions will be appropriate. The sample will include women over 65 years of age who have had surgery for breast cancer. The findings of the evaluation will not be applicable to women under age 65 with other types of cancer who have had only a diagnostic biopsy, have not had surgery, or have had bilateral mastectomy.

The independent variables are the evaluator's guide to determining where to set inclusion and exclusion criteria. For example, suppose that in an evaluation of the effects on teens of a language literacy program, one of the evaluation questions asks whether boys and girls benefit equally from program participation. In this question, the independent variable is gender, and the dependent (outcome) variable is benefit. If the evaluator plans to sample boys and girls, he or she must set inclusion and exclusion criteria.

Inclusion criteria for this evaluation might include boys and girls under 18 years old who are likely to attend all the educational activities for the duration of the evaluation and who are not able to read at levels appropriate for their ages. Teens might be excluded if they already participate in another language literacy program, if they do not speak English, or if their parents object to their participation. If these hypothetical inclusion and exclusion criteria are used to guide sampling eligibility, then the evaluation's findings can be generalized only to English-speaking boys and girls under age 18 who do not read appropriately for their age and tend to be compliant with school attendance requirements. The evaluation is not designed to enable the findings to be applicable to teens who have difficulty reading or speaking English and who are unlikely to be able to complete all program activities.

SAMPLING METHODS

Sampling methods are usually divided into two types: probability sampling and convenience sampling. Probability sampling is considered the best way to ensure the validity of any inferences made about a program's effectiveness and its generalizability. In probability sampling, every member of the target population has a known probability of being included in the sample.

In convenience sampling, participants are selected because they are available. Thus, in this kind of sampling, some members of the target population have a chance of being chosen whereas others do not even if they meet inclusion criteria. As a result, the data that is collected from a convenience sample may not be applicable at all to the target group.

For example, suppose an evaluator who is studying the quality of care provided by student health services decides to interview all students who come for care during the week of December 26. Suppose also that 100 students come, and all agree to be interviewed: a perfect response rate. The problem is that in some parts of the world, the end of December is associated with increased rates of illness from respiratory viruses as well as with high numbers of skiing accidents; moreover, many universities are closed during that week, and most students are not around. Thus, the data collected by the happy evaluator with the perfect response rate could very well be biased, because the evaluation excluded many students simply because they were not on campus and, if they were sick, might have received care elsewhere.

Simple Random Sampling

In simple random sampling, every subject or unit has an equal chance of being selected. Because of this equality of opportunity, random samples are considered relatively unbiased. Typical ways of selecting a simple random sample include applying a table of random numbers (available freely online) or a computer-generated list of random numbers to lists of prospective participants.

Suppose an evaluation team wants to select ten social workers at random from a list (or sampling frame) of 20 names. Each social worker is assigned an ID of 01 to 20. Using a table of random numbers (Table 4.1), the evaluators first identify a row of numbers at random and then a column. Where the two intersect, they begin to identify their sample.

This is how the evaluators obtained their sample.

1. *How they randomly identify the row:* A member of the evaluation team tosses a die twice. On the first toss, the die's number is 3; the number on the second toss is 5. Starting with the first column in the table, these numbers correspond to the third block and the fifth row of that block, or the row containing numbers 1 4 5 7 5 in Table 4.1.
2. *How they randomly identify the column:* A member of the team tosses the die twice and gets 2 and 1. Starting with the second column in the table these numbers correspond to the second block and the first row, which is 1 9 7 0 4. The starting point for this sample is where the row 1 4 5 7 5 and the column 1 9 7 0 4 intersect, at 3 5 4 9 0.
3. *How they select the sample:* The evaluators need ten social workers from their list of 20. Moving down from 3 5 4 9 0, the ten numbers between 01 and 20 that appear are 12, 20, 09, 01, 02, 13, 18, 03, 04, and 16. Social workers with these IDs are selected for the random sample.

Random Selection and Random Assignment

In any given evaluation, the process of random selection may be different from the process of random assignment, as is illustrated in Example 4.3.

Table 4.1 A Table of Random Numbers

1 8 2 8 3	1 9 7 0 4²	4 5 3 8 7	2 3 4 7 6	1 2 3 2 3	3 4 8 6 5
4 6 4 5 3	2 1 5 4 7	3 9 2 4 6	9 3 1 9 8	9 8 0 0 5	6 5 9 8 8
1 9 0 7 6	2 3 4 5 3	3 2 7 6 0	2 7 1 6 6	7 5 0 3 2	9 9 9 4 5
3 6 7 4 3	8 9 5 6 3	*1 2* 3 7 8	1 8 2 8 3	2 3 4 6 5	2 5 4 0 8
2 2 1 2 5	1 9 7 8 6	2 3 4 9 8	7 6 5 7 5	7 6 4 3 5	6 3 4 4 2
7 6 0 0 9	7 7 0 9 9	4 3 7 8 8	3 6 6 5 9	7 4 3 9 9	*0 3* 4 3 2
0 9 8 7 8	7 6 5 4 9	8 8 8 7 7	2 6 5 8 7	4 4 6 3 3	7 7 6 5 9
3 4 5 3 4	4 4 4 7 5	5 6 6 3 2	3 4 3 5 0	*0 1* 7 6 8	2 9 0 2 7
8 3 1 0 9	7 5 8 9 9	3 4 8 7 7	2 1 3 5 7	2 4 3 0 0	0 0 8 6 9
8 9 0 6 3	4 3 5 5 5	3 2 7 0 0	7 6 4 9 7	3 6 0 9 9	9 7 9 5 6
			9 4 6 5 6	3 4 6 8 9	
0 9 8 8 7	6 7 7 7 0	6 9 9 7 5	5 4 4 6 5	*1 3* 8 9 6	*0 4* 6 4 5
2 3 2 8 0	3 4 5 7 2	9 9 4 4 3	9 8 7 6 5	3 4 9 7 8	4 2 8 8 0
9 3 8 5 6	2 3 0 9 0	2 2 2 5 7	6 7 4 0 0	2 3 5 8 0	2 4 3 7 6
2 1 2 5 6	5 0 8 6 3	5 6 9 3 4	7 0 9 9 3	3 4 7 6 5	3 0 9 9 6
1 4 5 7 5¹	3 5 4 9 0³	2 3 6 4 5	2 2 1 7 9	3 5 7 8 8	3 7 6 0 0
2 3 2 7 6	7⁴ 0 8 7 0	*2 0* 0 8 7	6 6 6 6 5	7 8 8 7 6	5 8 0 0 7
8 7 5 3 0	4 5 7 3 8	*0 9* 9 9 8	4 5 3 9 7	4 7 5 0 0	3 4 8 7 5
0 0 7 9 1	3 2 1 6 4	9 7 6 6 5	2 7 5 8 9	9 0 0 8 7	*1 6* 0 0 4
9 9 0 0 3	3 2 5 6 7	*0 2* 8 7 8	3 8 6 0 2	*1 8* 7 0 0	2 3 4 5 5
1 4 3 6 7	6 4 9 9 9	7 8 4 5 3	4 0 0 7 8	5 3 7 2 7	2 8 7 5 9

[1] A member of the evaluation team tosses a die twice. On the first toss, the die's number is 3; the number on the second toss is 5. Starting with the first column in the table, these numbers correspond to the third block and the fifth row of that block, or the **row** containing numbers 1 4 5 7 5.
[2] A member of the team tosses the die twice and gets 2 and 1. Starting with the second column in the table, these numbers correspond to the second block and the first row, which is 1 9 7 0 4. The starting point for this sample is where the row 1 4 5 7 5 and the column beginning with 1 9 7 0 4 intersect, at 3 5 4 9 0.
[3] The intersection of 1 and 2.
[4] Start at 7 0 8 7 4 to get the sample.

Example 4.3 Random Selection and Random Assignment: Two Illustrations

Evaluation A

Evaluation A had six months to identify a sample of teens to participate in an evaluation of an innovative school-based preventive health care program. At the end of the six months, all eligible teens were assigned to the innovative program or the traditional (control) program. Assignment was based on how close to a participating school each teen lived. The evaluators used this method because participation meant that students would be required to attend several after-school activities, and no funding was available for transportation.

Evaluation B

Evaluation B had six months to identify a sample of teens to participate in an evaluation of an innovative school-based preventive health care program. At the end of the six months, a sample was randomly selected from the population of all teens who were eligible. Half the sample was randomly assigned to the innovative program, and half were assigned to the traditional (control) program.

In Evaluation A in this example, the evaluators selected all eligible teens and then assigned them to the experimental and control groups according to how close each one lived to a participating school. In Evaluation B, the evaluators selected a random sample of all those who were eligible and then randomly assigned the participants either to the experimental group or the control group. Of these two methods, the latter is usually considered preferable to the former. *Random selection* means that every eligible person has an equal chance of becoming part of the sample; if all are included because they just happen to appear during the time allocated for sampling, biases may be introduced. Random assignment can also guard against bias.

Systematic Sampling

Suppose an evaluator has a list with the names of 3,000 psychologists from which a sample of 500 is to be selected. In systematic sampling, the evaluator would divide 3,000 by 500 to yield 6, and then select every sixth name on the list. An alternative would be to select a number at random—say, by tossing a die. If the toss came up with the number 5, for example, the evaluator would select the fifth name on the list, then the tenth, the fifteenth, and so on, until he or she had the necessary 500 names.

Systematic sampling is not an appropriate method to use if repetition is a natural component of the sampling frame. For example, if the frame is a list of names, those beginning with certain letters of the alphabet (in English: Q or X) might get excluded because they appear infrequently.

Stratified Sampling

A *stratified random sample* is one in which the population is divided into subgroups, or *strata*, and a random sample is then selected from each group. For example, in a program to teach women of differing ages about options for the treatment of breast cancer, the evaluator might choose to sample women of differing general health status (as indicated by scores on a 32-item survey with 25 to 32 points meaning excellent and 1 to 8 meaning poor health status), age, and income (high, average, and low =). In this case, health status, age, and income are the strata. This sampling blueprint can be depicted as shown in Table 4.2.

Table 4.2 Sampling Blueprint for a Program to Educate Women in Options for Breast Cancer Treatment

Health Status Scores and Income	**Age (Years)**				
	< 35	35–55	56–65	66–75	> 75
25–32 points High income					
Average					
Low					
17–24 points High income					
Average					
Low					
9–16 points High income					
Average					
Low					
1–8 points High income					
Average					
Low					

To be meaningful, evaluators must select the strata or subgroups for the sample using justifiable criteria that link the independent variables (age, health status, and income) to the outcome (language literacy, convicted felon recidivism, breast cancer treatment choices). Justifiable criteria come from the research literature and expert opinion.

The strata in stratified sampling are subsets of the independent variables. If an independent variable is health status, the strata consist of how it is defined and measured—for example, excellent, good, fair, poor as measured by a validated survey. In Table 4.2, measurement of health status results in a score with 25 to 32 points equaling excellent and 1 to 8 points equaling poor health status.

If the evaluator does not use stratification in the choice of a sample, the results may be confounded. For example, if the evaluation fails to distinguish among women with different characteristics (age, health status, income), the outcomes (e.g., scores on a test) might be averaged among them, and the program might seem to have no overall effect even if women in one or more groups benefited. For example, the program might have been very successful with certain women, such as those under 35 years of age who have moderate incomes and health status scores between 25 and 32, but other women's average scores canceled the effect.

Statistical techniques (such as analysis of covariance and regression) can be used *retrospectively* (after the data has already been collected) to correct for confounders or covariates on the dependent variables or outcomes. Evaluators agree, however, that it is better to anticipate confounding variables than to correct for them after the fact through statistical analysis. Statistical corrections require very strict assumptions about the nature of the data, assumptions for which the sampling plan may not have been designed. With few exceptions, using statistical corrections afterward results in a loss of power, or the ability to detect true differences between groups (such as the experimental and control groups).

Cluster Sampling

Cluster sampling is used in large evaluations—those that involve many settings, such as universities, hospitals, cities, provinces, and so on. In cluster sampling, the population is divided into batches that are then randomly selected and assigned, and their constituents can be randomly selected and assigned. For example, suppose that California's counties are trying out a new program to improve emergency care for critically ill and injured children, and the control program is the traditional emergency medical system. If you want to use random cluster sampling to evaluate this program, you can consider each county to be a cluster and select and assign counties at random to the new program or the traditional program. Alternatively, you can randomly select children's hospitals and other facilities treating critically ill children within counties and randomly assign them to the experimental system or the traditional system (assuming this were considered ethical). Example 4.4 gives an illustration of the use of cluster sampling in a survey of Italian parents' attitudes toward AIDS education in their children's schools.

Example 4.4 Cluster Sampling in a Study of Attitudes of Italian Parents Toward AIDS Education

Epidemiologists from 14 of Italy's 21 regions surveyed parents of 725 students from 30 schools chosen by a cluster sampling technique from among the 292 classical, scientific, and technical high schools in Rome. Staff visited each school and selected students using a list of random numbers based on the school's size. Each of the students selected for participation was given a letter to deliver to his or her parents explaining the goals of the study and when they would be contacted.

Random sampling, no matter how complex, can be facilitated by using computer-generated randomized lists and online, sometimes proprietary, software applications.

Nonprobability or Convenience Sampling

Convenience samples are samples for which the probability of selection is unknown. Evaluators use convenience samples simply because they are easy to obtain. This means that some people have no chance of being selected simply because they are not around to be chosen. Convenience samples are more than likely to be biased, or not representative of the target population, unless proven otherwise.

In some cases, evaluators can perform statistical analyses to demonstrate that convenience samples are representative. For example, suppose that during the months of July and August, an evaluator conducts a survey of the needs of county institutions concerned with critically ill and injured children.

Because many county employees take their yearly vacations in July and August, the respondents may be different from those who would have answered the survey during other times of the year. If the evaluator wants to demonstrate that those employees who were around to respond and those who were not available in July and August are not different, he or she can compare the two groups on key variables, such as time on the job and experience with critically ill and injured children. If this comparison reveals no differences, the evaluator is in a relatively stronger position to assert that, even though the sample was chosen based on convenience, the characteristics of the participants do not differ on certain key variables (such as length of time on the job) from those of the target population.

THE SAMPLING UNIT

A major concern in sampling is the *unit* to be sampled. Example 4.5 illustrates the concept of the sampling unit.

Example 4.5 What Is the Target? Who Is Sampled?

An evaluation of a new program is concerned with measuring the program's effectiveness in altering physicians' practices pertaining to acute pain management for children who have undergone operations. The target population is all physicians who care for children undergoing operations.

The evaluation question is "Have physicians improved their pain management practices for children?" The evidence of effectiveness is that physicians in the experimental group show significant improvement over a one-year period and significantly greater improvement than physicians in a control group. Resources are available for 20 physicians to participate in the evaluation.

The evaluators will randomly assign ten physicians to the experimental group and ten physicians to the control. They plan to find out about pain management through a review of the medical records of ten patients of each of the physicians in the experimental and control groups, for a total sample of 200 patients. (This is sometimes called a *nested design.*)

A consultant to the evaluation team says that the evaluators are comparing the practices of ten physicians against those of ten physicians, and not the care of 100 patients against that of 100 patients. The reason is that characteristics of the care of the patients of any single physician will be highly related: They will cluster together. The consultant advises the evaluators to correct for this lack of "independence" among patients of the same physician by using one of the statistical methods available for correcting for cluster effects.

Another consultant, in contrast, advises the evaluators to use a much larger number of patients per physician and suggests a statistical method for selecting the appropriate number. Because the evaluators do not have enough money to enlarge the sample, they decide to "correct" statistically for the dependence among patients.

In this example, the evaluators want to be able to apply the evaluation's findings to all physicians who care for children undergoing surgery, but they have enough resources to include only 20 physicians in the evaluation. In an ideal world, the evaluators would have access to a very large number of physicians, but in the real world, they have only the resources to study ten patients per physician and access to statistical methods to correct for possible biases. These statistical methods enable evaluators to provide remedies for the possible dependence among the patients of a single physician, among students at a single institution, among health care workers at a single hospital, and so on.

SAMPLE SIZE

Power Analysis and Alpha and Beta Errors

An evaluation's ability to detect an effect is referred to as its *power*. A power analysis is a statistical method for identifying a sample size that will be large enough to allow the evaluator to detect an effect if one exists.

A commonly used evaluation research design is one in which the evaluator compares two randomly assigned groups to find out whether differences exist between them. "Does Program A differ from Program B in its ability to improve student's employability? self-confidence? reading ability?" is a typical generic evaluation question. To answer this question accurately, the evaluator must be sure that enough people are in each program group so that if a difference is present, it will be uncovered.

Conversely, if there is no difference between the two groups, the evaluator does not want to conclude falsely that there is one. To begin the process of making sure that the sample size is adequate to detect any true differences, the evaluator's first step is to reframe the appropriate evaluation questions into *null* hypotheses. Null hypotheses state that no difference exists between groups, as illustrated in Example 4.6.

Example 4.6 The Null Hypothesis

Question: Does Experimental Program A improve self-confidence?

Evidence: A statistically significant difference is found in self-confidence between Experimental Program A's participants and Control Program B's participants, and the difference is in Program A's favor.

Data source: The Self-Confidence Assessment, a 30-minute self-administered questionnaire with 100 questions. Scores on the Assessment range from 1 to 100, with 100 meaning highest self-confidence.

Null hypothesis: No difference in self-confidence exists between participants in Program A and participants in Program B. In other words, the average scores on the Self-Confidence Assessment obtained by participants in Program A and in Program B are equal.

When an evaluator finds that differences exist among programs but there are no differences, that is called an *alpha error* or *Type I error*. A Type I error is analogous to a false-positive test result—that is, a result indicating that a disease is present when it is not. When an evaluator finds that no differences exist among programs but differences actually do exist, that is termed a *beta error* or *Type II error*. A Type II error is analogous to a false-negative test result—that is, a result indicating that a disease is not present when it is. The relationship between what evaluators find and the true situation can be depicted as shown in Table 4.3.

Table 4.3 Type I and Type II Errors: Searching for the True Difference

		Truth	
		Differences Exist	**No Differences Exists**
Evaluators' conclusion from hypothesis test	**Differences exist (reject null)**	Correct	Type I or alpha error
	No differences exist (keep null)	Type II or beta error	Correct

To select sample sizes that will maximize the power of their evaluations, evaluators must rely on formulas whose use requires an understanding of hypothesis testing and a basic knowledge of statistics. Evaluators using these formulas usually must perform the following steps:

- State the null hypothesis.
- Set a level (alpha, or α) of statistical significance—usually .05 or .01—and decide whether it is to be a one- or two-tailed test.
- Decide on the smallest acceptable meaningful difference or effect (e.g., the difference in average scores between groups must be at least 15 points).
- Set the power $(1 - \beta)$ of the evaluation, or the chance of detecting a difference (usually 80% or 90%).
- Estimate the standard deviation (assuming that the distribution of the data is normal) in the population.

Some researchers have proposed alternative sample size calculations based on confidence intervals. A confidence interval is computed from sample data that has a given probability that the unknown parameter (such as the mean) is contained within the interval. Common confidence intervals are 90%, 95%, and 99%.

Calculating sample size is a technical activity that requires some knowledge of statistics. Several easy-to-use programs for calculating sample size are currently available for free online.

THE SAMPLING REPORT

Evaluators can use the sampling report (SR) form (Table 4.4) for planning and explaining their evaluations. The SR contains the evaluation questions and evidence, the independent variables and strata, the evaluation design, inclusion and exclusion criteria, the dependent variable, the data source, the criteria for level of acceptable statistical and practical (or educational or clinical) significance, the sampling methods, and the size of the sample.

The form in Table 4.4 shows the use of the SR for one evaluation question asked in an 18-month program combining diet and exercise to improve health status and quality of life for persons 65 years of age or older. An experimental group of elderly people who still live at home will receive the program and another group will not. To be eligible, participants must be able to live independently. People who are under 65 years of age and those who do not speak English or Spanish are not eligible.

Participants will be randomly assigned to the experimental or control groups according to the streets on which they live (i.e., participants living on Street A will be randomly assigned, as will participants living on Streets B, C, and so on). The evaluators will be investigating

Table 4.4 The Sampling Report Form

The Evaluation	The Report
Evaluation questions	1. To what extent has quality of life improved? 2. Do men and women differ in quality of life after participation?
Evidence of effectiveness	1. A statistical and practically meaningful difference between experimental and control group, favoring the experimental group. 2. Men and women benefit equally.
Evaluation design	An experimental design, with randomly assigned parallel controls.
Independent variables	Group participation; gender.
Strata	Group participation: experimental and control; gender: male and female.
Inclusion criteria	1. Must be living at home. 2. Must be functionally independent.
Exclusion criteria	1. Unable to speak English or Spanish. 2. 64 years of age or younger.
Dependent variable	Quality of life.
Data Source	Quality of Life Questionnaire: a 100-point survey. The Questionnaire's manual states that, when used with persons over 70 years of age, the standard deviation (a measure of how much the score "spreads" from the mean or average score) is 10 points.
Criterion for practical meaning (effect size)	A difference of at least 5 points on the Quality of Life Questionnaire between experimental and control, favoring the experimental group. Statistical significance (alpha) = .01; power is 80% (beta = .20).
Sampling method	For group assignment: cluster sampling. All streets in the town are eligible. All eligible persons in a given street are randomly assigned to the experimental or control group. For gender: An equal number of men and women will be randomly selected from all who are eligible; men and women will be randomly assigned to an experimental or a control group. No two participants will live on the same street.
Sample size	To compare men and women, a total of 188 people is needed: 94 men and 94 women; 47 of each will be assigned to the experimental or control groups.

whether the program effectively improves quality of life for men and women equally. A random sample of men and women will be selected from all who are eligible, but no two will live on the same street. Then men and women will be assigned at random to the experimental group or the control group.

SUMMARY AND TRANSITION TO THE NEXT CHAPTER ON COLLECTING PROGRAM EVALUATION INFORMATION

This chapter discussed the advantages and limitations of probability and convenience sampling and how to think about the sample unit and sample size. The next chapter discusses the evaluator's data collection choices.

EXERCISE: CHAPTER 4

Directions

For each of the following situations, choose the best sampling method from among these choices:

A. Simple random sampling
B. Stratified sampling
C. Cluster sampling
D. Systematic sampling
E. Convenience sampling

Situation 1

The Family Resources Center has 40 separate family counseling groups, each with about 30 participants. The director of the Center has noticed a decline in attendance rates and has decided to try out an experimental program to improve them. The program is very expensive, and the Center can afford to finance only a 250-person program at first. If the evaluator randomly selects individuals from among all group members, this will create friction and disturb the integrity of some of the groups. As an alternative, the evaluator has suggested a plan in which five of the groups—150 people—will be randomly selected to take part in the experimental program and five groups will participate in the control.

Situation 2

The Medical Center has developed a new program to teach patients about cardiovascular fitness. An evaluation is being conducted to determine how effective the program is with males and females of different ages. The evaluation design is experimental, with concurrent controls. In this design, the new and traditional cardiovascular programs are compared. About 310 people signed up for the winter seminar. Of these, 140 are between 45 and 60 years old, and 62 of these 140 were men. The remaining 170 are between 61 and 75 years old, and 80 of these are men. The evaluators randomly selected 40 persons from each of the four subgroups and randomly assigned every other person to the new program and the remainder to the old program.

Situation 3

A total of 200 social workers signed up for a continuing education program. Only 50 teachers from this group, however, are eligible to participate in an evaluation of the program's impact. The evaluator assigns each participant a number from 001 to 200 and, using a table, selects 50 names by moving down columns of three-digit random numbers and taking the first 50 numbers within the range 001 to 200.

REFERENCES AND SUGGESTED READINGS

Cohen, J. (1988). *Statistical power analysis for the behavioral sciences* (2nd ed.). Hillsdale, NJ: Lawrence Erlbaum.

Hulley, S.B., Cummings, S.R., Browner, W.S., Grady, D., Hearst, N., & Newman, T.B. (2022). *Designing clinical research* (5th ed.). Wolters Kluwer.

Example of Simple Randomization

Dehghan, N., Azizzadeh Forouzi, M., Etminan, A., Roy, C., & Dehghan M. (2022). The effects of lavender, rosemary and orange essential oils on memory problems and medication adherence among patients undergoing hemodialysis: A parallel randomized controlled trial. *Explore (New York, NY), 18*(5): 559–566.

Examples of a Cluster Sample

Faria, J.S., Marcon, S.R., Nespollo, A.M., et al. (2022). Attitudes of health professionals towards suicidal behavior: An intervention study. *Revista de saude publica, 56*: 54.

Kiviruusu, O., Björklund, K., Koskinen, H.L., et al. (2016). Short-term effects of the "Together at School" intervention program on children's socio-emotional skills: A cluster randomized controlled trial. *BMC Psychology, 4*(1): 27.

Examples of Stratified Random Sample

Leadbitter, K., Smallman, R., James, K., et al. (2022). REACH-ASD: A UK randomised controlled trial of a new post-diagnostic psycho-education and acceptance and commitment therapy programme against treatment-as-usual for improving the mental health and adjustment of caregivers of children recently diagnosed with autism spectrum disorder. *Trials, 23*(1): 585.

Saju, R., Castellon-Lopez, Y., Turk, N., et al. (2022). Differences in weight loss by race and ethnicity in the PRIDE trial: a qualitative analysis of participant perspectives. *Journal of General Internal Medicine, 37*(14): 3715–3722.

An Example of a Convenience Sample

Taillie, L.S., Prestemon, C.E., Hall, M.G., Grummon, A.H., Vesely, A., & Jaacks, L.M. (2022). Developing health and environmental warning messages about red meat: An online experiment. *PloS One, 17*(6): e0268121.

Suggested Websites

These websites provide definitions and explanations of sampling methods. For other sites, search for statistical sampling; how to sample; sampling methods; sampling strategies.

www.scribbr.com/methodology/sampling-methods

www.ncbi.nlm.nih.gov/pmc/articles/PMC4938277

https://s4be.cochrane.org/blog/2020/11/18/what-are-sampling-methods-and-how-do-you-choose-the-best-one

ANSWERS TO THE EXERCISE: CHAPTER 4

Situation 1: C
Situation 2: B
Situation 3: A

CHAPTER 5 | COLLECTING PROGRAM EVALUATION INFORMATION

PURPOSE OF CHAPTER 5

An evaluation's purpose is to produce unbiased information about a program's effectiveness, quality, and value. This chapter discusses evaluation information sources such as self-administered questionnaires (on and offline), achievement tests, database reviews, observations, interviews (in person, on the phone, online), and the literature. The advantages and limitations of each of these data sources are discussed as are their inherent sources of bias. This chapter also explains how to identify, search, and evaluate the published research literature because evaluators frequently rely on it to find useful data sources and measures.

A READER'S GUIDE TO CHAPTER 5

DOI: 10.4324/9781032635071-5

INFORMATION SOURCES: WHAT'S THE QUESTION?

An evaluator is asked to study the effectiveness of the At-Home Program, a program whose main objectives include providing high-quality health care and improving the health status and quality of life for elderly persons over 75 years of age who are still living at home. At-Home, the experimental program, consists of a comprehensive assessment of each elderly participant by an interdisciplinary team of health care providers and a home visit every three months by a nurse to monitor progress and reevaluate health and function. The control program consists of older people in the same communities who are not visited by the nurse and continue with their usual sources of care.

What information should the evaluator collect to find out whether the At-Home Program's objectives have been achieved? Where should the information come from? The evaluation questions and evidence of effectiveness and their associated independent and dependent variables provide answers. Consider the illustrations from the evaluation of the At-Home Program in Example 5.1.

Example 5.1 Evaluation Questions, Evidence, Variables, and Data Sources

Evaluation Question 1

Question: Has quality of care improved for diabetic patients in the At-Home and control program?
Evidence: A statistically and clinically meaningful improvement in quality of care is observed in experimental diabetic patients compared with control diabetic patients.
Independent variable: Group participation (experimental diabetics and control diabetics).
Potential sources of information to assign participants to groups: Physical examination, medical record review, surveys of health care practitioners and participants.
Dependent variable: Quality of care.
Potential sources of information to evaluate quality of care: Medical record review and surveys of health care practitioners and participants.

Evaluation Question 2

Question: Is quality of life improved for At-Home and control program participants? One aspect of good quality of life is the availability of a network of family and friends.
Evidence: A statistically significant difference between experimental and control programs in the availability of a network of family and friends.
Independent variable: Group participation (experimental and control).
Potential sources of information to assign participants to groups: Physical examination, medical record review, surveys of health care practitioners and participants.
Dependent variable: Availability of a network of family and friends.
Potential sources of information to assess the availability of a network of friends: Surveys of participants and their family members and friends, surveys of health care practitioners, observations.

To answer the first question in Example 5.1, the evaluator has at least two implicit tasks: identifying people with diabetes and assigning them to the experimental and control groups. People with diabetes can be identified through physical examination, medical record review, or surveys of health care practitioners and patients. Quality of care for diabetes can be measured through medical record review or through a survey of health care practitioners.

To identify people in the experimental and control groups for the second question in Example 5.1, the evaluator can examine the study's database. To measure the availability of each patient's network, the evaluator can survey patients, their friends, and family members.

Given the range of choices for each evaluation question, on what basis should the evaluator choose, say, to interview families rather than administer a questionnaire to the study's participants? How should the evaluator decide between medical record reviews and physical exams as data sources? Answering these questions is at the heart of a program evaluation's data collection.

CHOOSING APPROPRIATE DATA SOURCES

Evaluators have access to an arsenal of methods for collecting information. Among these are self-administered questionnaires (on- and offline performance and achievement tests), face-to-face and telephone interviews, observations, analysis of existing databases and vital statistics (such as infant mortality rates), the literature, and personal, medical, financial, and other statistical records. There are advantages and limitations to using each of these. To choose appropriate data sources for your program evaluation, you need to ask the following questions:

Guidelines: Questions to Ask in Choosing Data Sources

- What variables need to be measured? Are they defined and specific enough to measure?
- Can you borrow or adapt a currently available measure, or must you create a new one?
- If an available measure seems to be appropriate, has it been tried out in circumstances that are like those in which your evaluation is being conducted?
- Do you have the technical skills, financial resources, and time to create a valid measure?
- If no measure is available or appropriate, can you develop one in the time allotted for the evaluation?
- Do you have the technical skills, financial resources, and time to collect information with the chosen measure?
- Are participants likely to be able to fill out forms, answer questions, and provide information called for by the measure?
- In an evaluation that involves direct services to patients or students and uses information from medical, school, or other confidential records, can you obtain permission to collect data in an ethical way?
- To what extent will users of the evaluation's results (e.g., practitioners, students, patients, program developers, and sponsors) have confidence in the sources of information on which they are based?

Example 5.2 shows what can happen when evaluators neglect to answer these questions.

Example 5.2 (Not) Collecting Evaluation Information: A Case Study

The evaluators of an innovative third-year core surgery clerkship prepared a written examination to find out whether students learned to test donor–recipient compatibility before transfusion of red blood cells. The examination (to be given before and after the clerkship) included questions about the mechanisms involved in and consequences of transfusing incompatible red cells, the causes of incompatible transfusions, what to do about Rh-negative females who may bear children, how to identify unusual red cell antibodies, and what to do when no compatible blood is available.

The evaluators also planned to prepare a measure of students' understanding of ethical issues in blood transfusion that would consist of ten hypothetical scenarios with ethical components. They intended to compare students' responses to standards of ethics set by the University Blood Bank.

Finally, the evaluators anticipated distributing a self-administered survey to students before and after their participation in the clerkship to find out if their attitudes toward transfusion medicine changed. The results of the evaluators' activities were to be presented at a special meeting of the School of Medicine's Curriculum Committee one year after the start of the innovative program.

The evaluators' report turned out to be very brief. Although they were able to locate several achievement tests with questions about donor–recipient compatibility, and thus did not have to prepare these measures "from scratch," they could not find an appropriate time to give all students a pre-measure and post-measure. This meant that the evaluators had incomplete information on the performance of many students, with only pretests for some and only posttests for others. In addition, the evaluators found that developing the measure involving scenarios took about nine months because it was more difficult to create the scenarios than they had anticipated. A sample of students found the original scenarios hard to understand and ambiguous, so the evaluators had to rewrite and retest them. In the end, the scenario measure was not even ready for use at reporting time.

Finally, many students refused to complete the attitude questionnaire. Anecdotal information suggested that students felt they were overloaded with tests and questionnaires and that they did not believe this additional one was important. Because of the poor quality of the data, the evaluators were unable to provide any meaningful information about the third-year surgery clerkship's effectiveness.

In the case presented above, the evaluators encountered difficulties for three major reasons:

1. They did not have enough time to collect data on students' achievement before and after.
2. They did not have enough time and possibly lacked the skills to prepare the scenarios for a planned measure.
3. They chose a method of information collection that was not appropriate for the participants as demonstrated by their unwillingness to complete it.

SOURCES OF DATA IN PROGRAM EVALUATION AND THEIR ADVANTAGES AND LIMITATIONS

Self-Administered Surveys

In self-administered surveys (or questionnaires), respondents answer questions or respond to items, on paper or online. Self-administered surveys in hard-copy form (whether distributed through the mail, in a classroom or clinic, or in some other way) differ from online surveys in who does the scoring and data entry. The responses that participants fill in on paper questionnaires must be scanned or entered into a database by hand for statistical analysis. Online survey responses are automatically entered and can provide the evaluator instantly with information about the number of respondents, who they are demographically, and how many questionnaires were completed.

Online surveys are efficient because they save paper, can be completed anywhere, save the time needed for data entry with paper surveys (and the errors that may go with it), and do away with the need to find storage space for and protection of completed paper forms. Moreover, mailed surveys, one source of self-administered surveys, are becoming increasingly impossible to rely on in many parts of the world where posted mail is infrequent or unreliable. However, online surveys are not always possible either because not all areas of the world have reliable internet access or mobile phone reception.

To maximize the efficiency of online surveys, evaluators must be sure they have the technical expertise necessary to prepare and advertise online questionnaires and ensure respondent privacy. Because of the strict rules regarding participant privacy, evaluators using online surveys may need to acquire dedicated computers or tablets and set up firewalls and other protections.

Self-Administered Survey Questionnaire Advantages

- Many people are accustomed to completing questionnaires, regardless of where or how they are administered.
- Many questions and rating scales are available for adaptation.
- Online questionnaires can reach large groups of people at relatively low cost.
- Online surveys produce immediate findings.

Self-Administered Survey Questionnaire Disadvantages

- Survey respondents may not always tell the truth.
- The self-administered survey format is not suitable for obtaining explanations of behavior.
- Some respondents may fail to answer some or even all questions, leaving the evaluator with incomplete information.
- Some people ignore unsolicited online surveys because they think they receive too many requests. Advanced planning is essential to ensure that your survey is not automatically deleted or put into spam or junk mail.

Tests

A test is a series of questions or practical exercises for measuring the skill, knowledge, intelligence, capacities, or aptitudes of an individual or group.

Tests are frequently used in evaluations to measure individuals' knowledge and understanding of facts, their ability to apply theories and principles, and their capacity for innovation. To assess higher levels of learning, such as the evaluation of evidence or the synthesis of information from varying sources, other methods (such as observation of performance or analysis of essays, works of art, and scientific studies) may be more appropriate.

Other tests used in evaluations include medical tests such as pregnancy or vision tests and mental health tests for depression or anxiety.

Database Reviews

Database reviews are analyses of documented or recorded behavior and events. The documents may be in print, audio, or video form.

Databases come in two formats. The first consists of already existing records (school attendance data, morbidity and mortality statistics, data on prison occupancy). The second database format is comprised of data collected primarily for the evaluation. For example, in an evaluation of a program to improve how students use research information online, the evaluators might use achievement tests and satisfaction surveys. Data from the two information sources will constitute the evaluation's database.

Existing Databases

Evaluators use data from existing databases because doing so reduces the burden that occurs when people are required to complete surveys or achievement tests. Existing records are *unobtrusive measures*. Why ask people to spend their time answering questions when the answers are already available? Birth date, gender, place of birth, and other demographic variables are often found in accessible records and need not be asked directly of people.

Existing databases are also relatively accurate sources of data on behavior. For example, evaluators interested in the effects of a program on school attendance can ask students, teachers, or parents about attendance. But school records are probably more reliable because they do not depend on people's recall, and they are updated regularly. For the same reason, records are also good places to find out about actual practices. Which treatments are usually prescribed? Check a sample of medical records. How many foster children were adopted by their foster families? Check the foster agency files.

Existing databases are not always easily accessible, and so evaluators should be cautious in relying upon them. If an evaluator plans to use records from more than one site (e.g., two hospitals or four schools), the evaluation team may first have to learn how to access the data in each system and then create a mechanism for linking the data across them. This learning process can take time, and it may be costly.

Existing Database Advantages

- Obtaining data from existing records can be relatively unobtrusive because daily activities in schools, prisons, clinics, and so on need not be disturbed.
- Records are often a relatively reliable storehouse of actual practice or behavior.
- If data is needed on demographic characteristics such as age, gender, or insurance status, records are often the most reliable source.
- Data obtained from records eliminates participants' research burden.

Existing Database Disadvantages

- Finding information in records is often time-consuming. The evaluator may have to learn how to use multiple systems and go through an elaborate process to gain access to them.
- Reviews can vary from reviewer to reviewer. To ensure consistency, each record reviewer needs to be trained, and more than one reviewer is recommended. The costs of not having to collect new data may be offset by other expenses.
- Certain types of information are not always recorded such as how people behave, feel, or perceive.
- Records do not provide data on the appropriateness of a practice or on the relationship between what was done (process) and results (outcomes and impact).

Large Databases, a Special Kind of Existing Database

Evaluators often use large databases to help program planners to explore the need for new programs and to set evaluation standards by studying previous performance. Does the data show that students are underperforming in math? Perhaps a new program is needed. Is every eligible patient receiving flu shots? Perhaps the existing program needs improvement.

Large databases are useful in observational evaluations. For example, an evaluator can use a school's statistics database to compare students who participated last year in Programs A and B. Did Program A improve attendance as hoped?

Observational evaluations may require the creation of separate data sets. A data set is a new database that is a subset of a larger one. Suppose a database contains information on students in

Programs A, B, and C. The evaluator who wants to compare students only in Programs A and B will have to create a separate dataset that contains information on just the needed students and programs.

The analysis of data from existing databases is called *secondary data analysis*. Tutorials for using U.S. and other health databases like the ones maintained by the U.S. Census and the World Health Organization are available at:

www.nlm.nih.gov/nichsr/stats_tutorial/section4/ex1_NCHS.html

Statistical information and access to data on education in the U.S. are available at the National Center for Education Statistics, https://nces.ed.gov.

Evaluators use secondary data from large databases because it is comparatively economical to do so. Although professional skill is needed in creating data sets and analyzing data, the costs in time and money are probably less than the resources needed to do *primary data* collection. Primary data is collected by evaluators to meet the specific needs of their project.

Large Database Advantages

- Sometimes primary data collection is simply not necessary because the available data solves the problem or answers the question.
- Using existing data can be less expensive and time-consuming than collecting new data.
- Secondary sources of information can yield more accurate data for some variables than can primary sources. For instance, data collected by governments or international agencies from surveys tends to be accurate. The data collection methods and processes are often perfected over time with large numbers of people.
- Secondary data is especially useful in the exploratory phase of large studies or program planning efforts. They can be used to determine the prevalence of a problem, and to study if certain members of a given population are more susceptible to the problem than others.

Large Database Disadvantages

- The definitions of key variables that the original data collectors use may be different from yours. Definitions of terms like quality of life or self-efficacy may vary considerably from time to time and country to country, for example.
- The information in the database may not be presented exactly as you need it. The original researchers collected information on people's health behaviors in the past year, for example, but you need data on those behaviors in last month. The original researchers asked for categorical responses (often, sometimes, rarely), but you want continuous data (number of drinks per day; scores on a test).
- The data in the database may have come from a community that is somewhat different from yours in age, socioeconomic status, health behaviors, social work and education policies, etc.
- The reliability of published statistics can vary over time. Systems for collecting data change. Geographical or administrative boundaries are changed by government, or the basis for stratifying a sample is altered.
- Available data may be out of date by the time you gain access to the database. Large databases are typically updated periodically—say, every five years. This time lag may acquire significance if new policies are put in place between the time of the original data collection and the evaluator's access.

Observations

Observations are a form of data collection in which the evaluator collects data either in person or by way of a camera. Observations are appropriate for describing the environment (e.g., the size of a classroom, the number of pictures on a wall) and for obtaining global portraits of the dynamics of a situation (e.g., a typical problem-solving session among teachers or a "day in the life" of a school).

Observation Advantages

- Observations provide evaluators with an opportunity to collect firsthand information.
- Observations may provide evaluators with information that they did not anticipate collecting. For instance, when reviewing closed-circuit TV placed in a classroom, they may find that some children consistently do not participate in group activities.

Observation Disadvantages

- Evaluation personnel must receive extensive training and follow a very structured format to collect reliable observations.
- The process of observation is both labor-intensive and time-consuming.
- Observers can influence the environment they are studying, and observed individuals may behave differently than they might otherwise because they are being watched.

Interviews

Interviews are used in evaluations to speak directly to participants. Interviews can be conducted in person, online, or over the phone.

Interview Advantages

- Interviews allow the evaluator to ask participants about the meanings of their answers.
- Interviews can be useful for collecting information from people who may have difficulty reading or seeing.

Interview Disadvantages

- The process of conducting interviews is both time-consuming and labor-intensive.
- Interviewers must receive extensive training before they begin interviewing, and their work must be monitored on an ongoing basis.
- Interviewers may need special skills to interpret responses that are "off the record."

Computer-Assisted Interviews

With computer-assisted telephone interviewing or CATI, the interviewer reads instructions and questions to the respondent directly from a computer monitor and enters the responses directly into the computer. The computer, not the interviewer, controls the progression of the interview questions.

CATI software programs enable the researcher to enter all telephone numbers and call schedules into the computer. When an interviewer logs on, he or she is prompted with a list of phone numbers to call, including new scheduled interviews and callbacks. For example, suppose the interviewer calls someone at 8:00 a.m. but receives no answer. The CATI program can automatically reschedule the call for some other time. CATI programs are also available that enable specially trained interviewers to contact respondents with unique needs. For instance, suppose your evaluation sample consists of people who speak different languages. CATI allows multilingual interviewers to log on with certain keywords; the computer then directs them to their unique set of respondents.

CATI takes two forms. In one, the interviews are conducted from a lab, a facility furnished with banks of telephone calling stations equipped with computers linked to a central server. The costs of building such a lab, which must have soundproof cubicles and either a master computer that stores the data from the individual computers or linkage to a server, are extremely high.

Additional resources are needed to cover the cost of leasing CATI software and hiring a programmer to install it. Training for this type of CATI is expensive because the interviewers require a great deal of practice. Numerous incidental costs are also associated with establishing a CATI lab, including those for headsets, seats and desks, instructional manuals, and service contracts for the hardware.

The second type of CATI system uses software programs that are run on laptops or tablets. With this type of CATI, the evaluator needs only a laptop and wireless connection. This type of CATI is appropriate for studies with a variety of funding levels because it is portable and relatively inexpensive.

The portability of laptops and tablets, however, raises concerns about privacy. Laptops and tablets are sometimes shared or stolen, either of which can endanger the confidentiality of participant data. In anticipation of these concerns, evaluators who use laptops or tablets for CATI should dedicate them to a single study, enforce strict privacy safeguards, and offer interviewers special training to ensure proper CATI implementation and privacy protection.

The Research Literature

Evaluators turn to the literature for reasons that range from gathering ideas for research designs and data collection and analysis methods to comparing data and conclusions across research. The broad term *literature* refers to all published and unpublished reports of studies that pertain to the program and its methods, findings, and conclusions.

Published reports are easier to locate than those that remain unpublished, given that they have appeared in books and journals that are accessible online or in print from evaluation sponsors including governmental and non-governmental organizations and agencies. In addition, because published reports have the advantage of public scrutiny, their authors' methods (and the conclusions they have drawn) are likely to be more dependable. Reports on evaluation studies may be published in peer-reviewed journals, in books, or as stand-alone reports or monographs.

Program evaluators generally use the literature for the following reasons.

Guidelines for Reviewing the Literature

As an evaluator, you should take the following four steps in conducting a literature review:

1. Select relevant bibliographic databases.
2. Use precise terms and filters for the search.
3. Assemble the "best" literature available.
4. Extract the information.

Select Relevant Bibliographic Databases

There are hundreds of databases, online libraries, and open access journals that may contain literature that an evaluator will find to be useful. Some databases provide free access to their content (PubMed and the Educational Resources Information Center or ERIC, both of which are U.S. government sponsored), while access to others requires paid membership (PsycInfo, Web of Science). You can find a list of databases by searching online or by asking an LLM (large language model) or artificial intelligence (AI) program to help you. Another option is to identify one or more literature reviews in your field to see what databases are used. Evaluators often check several databases to be sure their review is complete.

Reasons for Evaluators' Use of the Literature

1. *To identify and justify evidence of effectiveness, quality, and value.* The literature can provide information on the past performance of programs and populations. Evaluators may use this information in planning an evaluation and as a yardstick against which to compare the findings of one that has already been completed.
2. *To define variables.* The literature is a primary source of information about the ways others have defined and measured commonly used key variables, such as child abuse and neglect; high-risk social and health behaviors; comorbid conditions; social, physical, and emotional functioning; quality of care; and quality of life.
3. *To determine sample size.* Power calculations, which evaluators use to arrive at sample sizes that are large enough to reveal true differences in programs (if they exist), require estimation of the variance—a measure of dispersion—in the sample or population. Sometimes, however, evaluators have no readily available data on the variance in the sample of interest. They can conduct a pilot study to obtain the data, but such studies are expensive, and appropriate data may be available in the literature.
4. *To obtain examples of designs, measures, and ways of analyzing and presenting data.* Evaluators can use the literature as a source of information on research methods and data collection, analysis, and reporting techniques.
5. *To determine the significance of the evaluation and its findings.* Evaluators use the literature to justify the need for programs and for their evaluation questions. They also use the literature to show whether their evaluation findings confirm or contradict the results of other studies and to identify areas in which little or no knowledge is currently available.
6. *To conduct meta-analyses.* Meta-analysis is a statistical technique in which the results of two or more randomized controlled trials are pooled and reanalyzed. The idea is that by combining the results of relatively small, local studies, one can increase the power of the findings. The use of meta-analysis is predicated on data from experimental studies, especially randomized controlled trials. Given that not all experiments are of equal quality, even RCTs, understanding how to review and interpret the literature is an important first step in conducting a meta-analysis.

Use Precise Terms and Filters for the Search

Searches using internet-based data are more efficient if the search terms are precise and the results are filtered by study and publication characteristics. Suppose you are interested in reviewing evaluations of child abuse prevention programs. If you go to PubMed, where you are likely to find information on child abuse, and enter the search terms, "program evaluation and child abuse prevention," you will get something like the results depicted in Figure 5.1.

This search results in 827 articles in June 2023. Reviewing this large number of articles is not only infeasible, but it is also more than likely to be unnecessary. Suppose, for example, you are only interested in full-text articles that describe the results of randomized controlled trials that have been published in the past five years. A more precise search with these filters shortens the list to 21 articles! (Figure 5.2).

The number of citations can be made even more relevant by adding additional filters. For example, adding a language (English) and an age filter (adolescents between 13 and 18) reduces the number of available full-text randomized controlled trials to 2! (Figure 5.3).

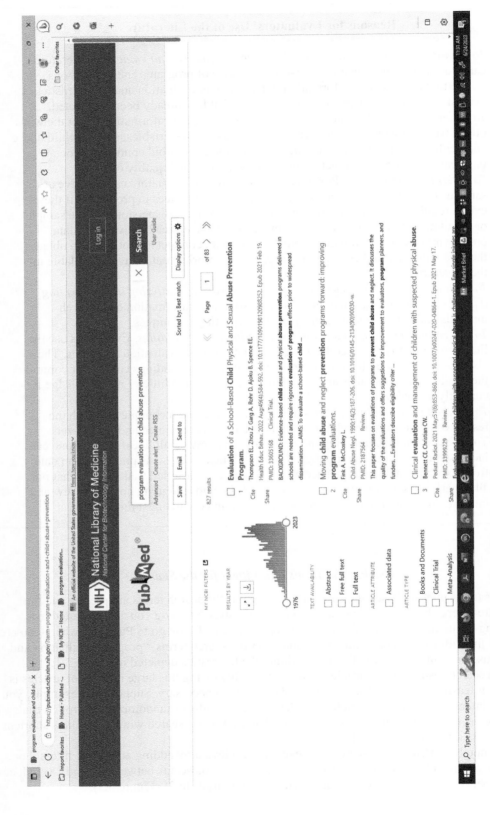

Figure 5.1 Using PubMed to Find Evaluations of Programs to Prevent Child Abuse

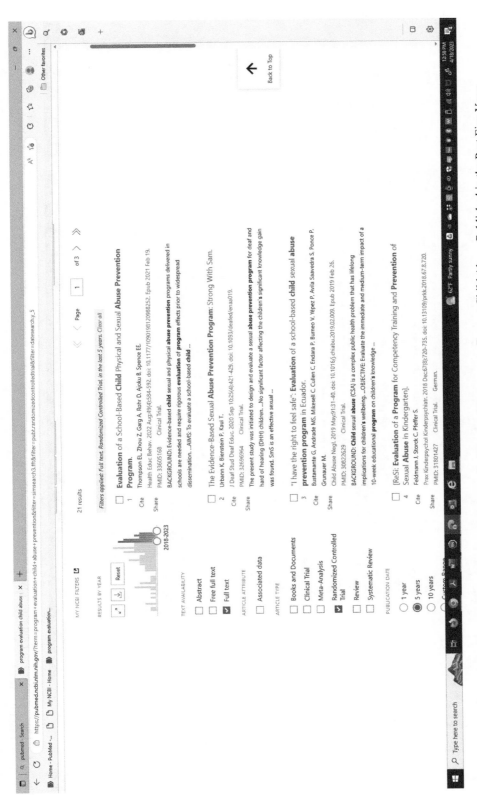

Figure 5.2 Using PubMed to Find Full-Text Randomized Controlled Trials of Programs to Prevent Child Abuse Published in the Past Five Years

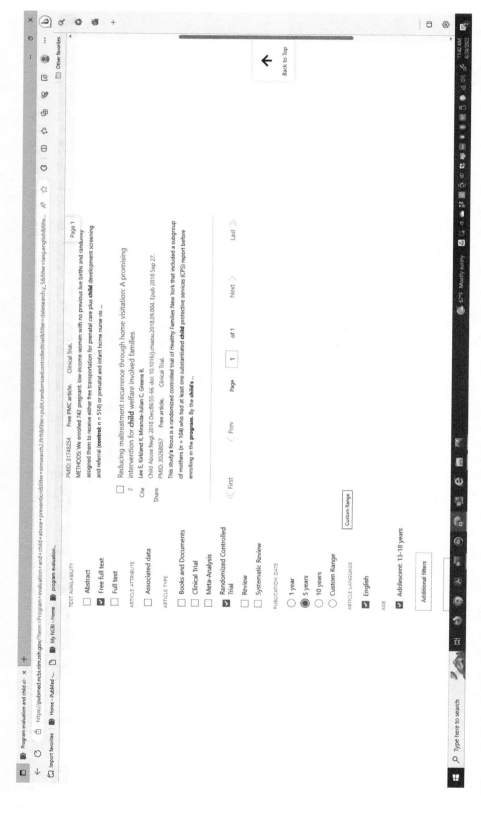

Figure 5.3 Using PubMed to Find Full-Text Randomized Controlled Trials of Programs to Prevent Child Abuse in Adolescents 13–18 Years Published in the Past Five Years

Rating Methodological Features of the Literature: Identifying the Best Published Prenatal Care Program Evaluations

Criteria for Selecting the Best Available Literature

- Description of the experimental program is clear (data is given on program's duration, funding level, services, providers, patients, standardization across sites, and so on).
- Participants are randomly selected for the evaluation (all patients are selected or a random sampling).
- Participants are randomly assigned to groups.
- Data collected for the evaluation is demonstrated to be valid for all main variables.
- The study focuses on outcomes (e.g., birth weight, gestational age, drug status of mother and baby).
- The study collects more than one measurement after participants complete the program.
- Statistical information is sufficient to determine the clinical and practical significance of the findings (e.g., confidence intervals, exact p values).

Assemble the "Best" Literature Available

Few searches (or searchers) are perfect, and they invariably turn up studies that do not address the topic of interest, are poorly designed, or are not current. Often, a brief review of the summary or abstract can help eliminate many irrelevant articles.

Identifying the best literature requires more effort. It means applying a set of criteria to make sure that the literature you eventually review is high quality and worth the effort of reviewing. Among the quality criteria you should consider are the robustness of the research design and the validity of the data collection measures.

The box below gives an example of methodological criteria that can be used in appraising the quality of the published literature.

The evaluator must decide how to score each potentially reviewable study: Does it have to meet all the criteria or some fraction (say, a score of more than 5 of 8), or does it have to achieve certain minimum criteria (such as random assignment and valid data collection)? These choices are somewhat arbitrary, and the evaluator must be able to defend their merits on a case-by-case basis.

Extract the Information

The most efficient way to get data from the literature is to standardize the review process. A uniform extraction system guards against the possibility that some important information will be missed, ignored, or misinterpreted. Extraction on forms often look like survey questionnaires as in Example 5.3.

Example 5.3 Excerpts from a Form to Guide Reviewers in Extracting Literature on Alcohol Misuse in Older Adults

1. Are main variables defined? (Circle one)
   No. . . . . .1 (*Go to Question 3*)
   Yes. 2

1a. If yes, please give definitions in authors' own words.

Term	Definition (if given by authors)
Alcoholism	
Heavy drinking	
Problem drinking	
Alcohol abuse	
Alcohol dependence	
Alcohol-related problems	

2. Describe the participating sample.

	65 to 74 Years of Age (n =)	75 Years of Age and Older (n =)
Male		
Female		
Other		
Total		

3. Are reasons given for incomplete or no data on eligible participants? (Check all that apply)

No. . . . . 1 *(Go to next question)*
Yes. 2

3a. If yes, what are they?

Incorrect address	❏
Medical problems; specify: _____	❏
Failure to show for an appointment	❏
Other; specify: _____	❏

4. Which of the following variables are explored in the study? (Check all that apply)

Quantity of alcohol consumed	❏
Frequency of alcohol consumed	❏
Medication use	❏
Health problems	❏
Functional status	❏
Symptoms	❏

5. For each variable included in the study, summarize the results and conclusions.

Variables	Summary of Results	Conclusions

Consider (but Be Careful with) the Non-Peer-Reviewed Literature

Various analyses of the published literature have suggested the existence of a bias in favor of positive results. This means that if your review is based solely on published, peer-reviewed evaluations, negative findings may be underrepresented. It is not easy, however, to locate and gain access to unpublished evaluation reports. Published studies have been reviewed by experts as well as the evaluator's peers and colleagues, and probably the most unreliable have been screened out. Nevertheless, when you are interpreting the findings from the published literature, you should consider the potential biases that may exist because unpublished reports are excluded. Unpublished reports include monographs, dissertations, blogs, and professional research sites. Statistical methods are available to account for publication bias. They are controversial, however, partly because they may create false positives (finding a benefit when none exists) under some circumstances.

SUMMARY AND TRANSITION TO THE NEXT CHAPTER ON EVALUATION MEASURES

This chapter has explained the factors that the evaluator should consider when deciding on measures or sources of data. First, the evaluator must carefully review the evaluation question so that all variables are known and clarified. Then the evaluator considers the array of possible measures that are likely to provide information on each variable. Among the possibilities are self-administered questionnaires, achievement and performance tests, database reviews, observations and interviews, physical examinations, and literature reviews.

Each data source or measure has advantages and disadvantages. For example, interviews enable the evaluator to question program participants in a relatively in-depth manner but conducting them can be time-consuming and costly. Self-administered questionnaires may be less time-consuming and costly than interviewers, but they lack the intimacy of interviews, and the evaluator must always worry about response rate.

In selecting a source of data for your evaluation, you must look first at the evaluation question and decide whether you have the technical and financial resources and the time to develop your own measure; if not, you must consider adopting or adapting an already existing measure.

The next chapter addresses the concepts of *reliability* (the consistency of the information from each source) and *validity* (the accuracy of the information). The chapter also discusses the steps you need to take to develop and validate your own measure and outlines the activities involved in selecting or adapting a measure that has been developed by other evaluators.

Among the additional topics addressed in the next chapter are "coding"—that is, making sure that your measure is properly formatted or described from the point of view of others who want to enter your data into another database for their own evaluations or better understand the data. For instance, is a high score coded "1," or is a low score coded "1? A measurement chart is presented that is helpful for portraying the logical connections among the evaluation's variables and measures.

EXERCISE: CHAPTER 5

Directions

Locate the following evaluations and name the types of measures used in each.

A. Chung, Y., & Huang, H.H. (2021). Cognitive-based interventions break gender stereotypes in kindergarten children. *International Journal of Environmental Research and Public Health*, *18*(24): 13052. https://doi.org/10.3390/ijerph182413052.

B. King, C.A., Kramer, A., Preuss, L., Kerr, D.C.R., Weisse, L., & Venkataraman, S. (2006). Youth-nominated support team for suicidal adolescents (version 1): A randomized controlled trial. *Journal of Consulting and Clinical Psychology*, *74*(1): 199–206. https://doi.org/10.1037/0022-006x.74.1.199.

C. Garrow, D., & Egede, L.E. (2006). Association between complementary and alternative medicine use, preventive care practices, and use of conventional medical services among adults with diabetes. *Diabetes Care*, *29*(1), 15–19. https://doi.org/10.2337/diacare.29.01.06.dc05-1448.

REFERENCES AND SUGGESTED READINGS

Examples of Literature Reviews

Bailey, E.J., Kruske, S.G., Morris, P.S., Cates, C.J., & Chang, A.B. (2008). Culture-specific programs for children and adults from minority groups who have asthma [Review]. *Cochrane Database of Systematic Reviews*, 8(8): CD006580.

Fink, A. (2019). *Conducting research literature reviews: From the internet to paper*. Thousand Oaks, CA: Sage.

Fink, A., Parhami, I., Rosenthal, R.J., Campos, M.D., Siani, A., & Fong, T.W. (2012). How transparent is behavioral intervention research on pathological gambling and other gambling-related disorders? A systematic literature review. *Addiction*, *107*(11): 1915–1928.

Hoffler, T.N., & Leutner, D. (2007). Instructional animation versus static pictures: A meta-analysis. *Learning and Instruction*, *17*(6): 722–738.

Hofmann, S.G., & Smits, J.A. (2008). Cognitive-behavioral therapy for adult anxiety disorders: A meta-analysis of randomized placebo-controlled trials. *Journal of Clinical Psychiatry*, *69*(4): 621–632.

Lemstra, M., Neudorf, C., D'Arcy, C., Kunst, A., Warren, L.M., & Bennett, N.R. (2008). A systematic review of depressed mood and anxiety by SES in youth aged 10–15 years. *Canadian Journal of Public Health*, *99*(2): 125–129.

Nigg, J.T., Lewis, K., Edinger, T., & Falk, M. (2012). Meta-analysis of attention-deficit/hyperactivity disorder or attention-deficit/hyperactivity disorder symptoms, restriction diet, and synthetic food color additives. [Article]. *Journal of the American Academy of Child and Adolescent Psychiatry*, *51*(1): 86–97. doi:10.1016/j.jaac.2011.10.015.

Prugger, J., Derdiyok, E., Dinkelacker, J., Costines, C., & Schmidt, T.T. (2022). The Altered States Database: Psychometric data from a systematic literature review. *Scientific Data*, *9*(1): 720.

Phoo, N.N.N., Lobo, R., Vujcich, D., & Reid, A. (2022). Comparison of the ACASI mode to other survey modes in sexual behavior surveys in Asia and Sub-Saharan Africa: Systematic literature review. *Journal of Medical Internet Research*, 24(5): e37356.

Pati, D., & Lorusso, L.N. (2018). How to write a systematic review of the literature. *HERD*, 11(1): 15–30.

Reynolds, S., Wilson, C., Austin, J., & Hooper, L. (2012). Effects of psychotherapy for anxiety in children and adolescents: A meta-analytic review. *Clinical Psychology Review*, *32*(4): 251–262. doi:10.1016/j.cpr.2012.01.005.

Shor, E., Roelfs, D.J., Bugyi, P., & Schwartz, J.E. (2012). Meta-analysis of marital dissolution and mortality: Reevaluating the intersection of gender and age. *Social Science & Medicine*, *75*(1): 46–59. doi:10.1016/j.socscimed.2012.03.010

Siegenthaler, E., Munder, T., & Egger, M. (2012). Effect of preventive interventions in mentally ill parents on the mental health of the offspring: Systematic review and meta-analysis. [Review]. *Journal of the American Academy of Child and Adolescent Psychiatry*, *51*(1): 8–17. doi:10.1016/j.jaac.2011.10.018.

Wiemker, V., Neufeld, M., Bunova, A., et al. (2022). Digital assessment tools using animation features to quantify alcohol consumption: Systematic app store and literature review. *Journal of Medical Internet Research*, *24*(3): e28927.

Wood, S., & Mayo-Wilson, E. (2012). School-based mentoring for adolescents: A systematic review and meta-analysis. [Review]. *Research on Social Work Practice*, *22*(3). doi:10.1177/1049731511430836.

Suggested Websites

National Library of Medicine: Finding and Using Health Statistics
www.nlm.nih.gov/oet/ed/stats/04-100.html

National Center for Education Statistics
https://nces.ed.gov

ANSWERS TO THE EXERCISE: CHAPTER 5

A. Chung and Huang

Picture classification task to measure gender stereotypes.

B. King and colleagues

The Suicidal Ideation Questionnaire—Junior is a 15-item self-report questionnaire used to assess the frequency of a wide range of suicidal thoughts.

The Spectrum of Suicide Behavior Scale is a five-point rating of the history of suicidality (none, ideation, intent/threat, mild attempt, serious attempt).

Measures of internalizing symptoms include the Youth Self-Report (YSR) internalizing scale and the Reynolds Adolescent Depression Scale (RADS). The YSR consists of 119 problem behavior items that form internalizing and externalizing scales. The RADS is a 30-item self-report questionnaire that assesses frequency of depressive symptoms on a four-point scale with endpoints of almost never and most of the time.

The CAFAS, Child and Adolescent Functional Assessment Scale, assesses functional impairment in multiple areas, including moods/self-harm. On the basis of parent responses to a structured interview, a trained clinician rates level of functioning on a four-point scale (0, 10, 20, 30) ranging from 0 (minimal or no impairment) to 30 (severe impairment).

C. Garrow and Egede

The 2002 National Health Interview Survey (NHIS), a national household survey sponsored by the National Center for Health Statistics, was used to collect data on whether participants had a diagnosis of diabetes or other illness, the use of complementary and alternative medicine, demographic and socioeconomic characteristics, preventive health care practices, and the use of conventional medical services.

CHAPTER 6 | EVALUATION MEASURES

An evaluation's data sources or measures include surveys, achievement tests, observations, database or record reviews, and interviews. Reliable and valid measures are the foundation of unbiased evaluation information. A reliable measure is consistent in its findings, and a valid one is accurate. This chapter discusses measurement validity in detail. It also explains how to develop reliable and valid new measures, select appropriate measures among those that are currently available, and create a measurement chart to establish logical connections among the evaluation's questions and hypotheses, design, and measures.

A READER'S GUIDE TO CHAPTER 6

DOI: 10.4324/9781032635071-6

RELIABILITY AND VALIDITY

A measure is the specific data source or *instrument* that evaluators use to collect data. For instance, the 25-item Open City Online Survey of Educational Achievement is a measure. The data source or data collection method is an online survey.

The term *metric* is sometimes used to describe how a concept is measured. For instance, to measure the school library's usefulness, an evaluator may ask patrons to use a rating scale with choices ranging from 1 (not useful) to 5 (extremely useful), or the evaluator may ask librarians to count the number of people who use the library over a two-year period. In the first example, the metric is a rating scale, and in the second, the metric is a count. Data collection measures take several formats (self-administered questionnaires or face-to-face interviews) and rely on a variety of metrics (rating scales, ranks).

Evaluators sometimes create their own measures, and sometimes they adapt or adopt parts or all of already existing ones. Because the conclusions of an evaluation are based on data from the measures used, the quality of the measures must be demonstrably high for the evaluation's results to be unbiased. (Otherwise, we have the well-known phenomenon of "garbage in— garbage out.") To determine the quality of their data collection measures, evaluators must understand the concepts of reliability and validity.

RELIABILITY

A *reliable* measure is one that is relatively free of "measurement error," which causes individuals' obtained scores to be different from their true scores (which can be obtained only through perfect measures).

What causes measurement error? In some cases, it results from the measure itself, as when the measure is difficult to understand or poorly administered. For example, a self-administered questionnaire regarding the value of preventive health care can produce unreliable results if it requires a level of reading ability that is beyond that of the teen mothers who are to use it. If the respondents' reading level is not a problem but the directions are unclear, the measure will also be unreliable. Unfortunately, the evaluator can simplify the measure's language and clarify the directions and still find measurement error because it can come directly from the people being questioned. If the teen mothers who are asked to complete a questionnaire are especially anxious or fatigued at the time, for example, their obtained scores might suffer and be quite different from their true, unbiased score.

In program evaluation, four kinds of reliability are often discussed: test-retest, equivalence, homogeneity, and inter- and intrarater reliability.

Test-Retest Reliability

A measure has *test-retest reliability* if the correlation between scores on the measure from one time to another is high. Suppose a survey of social service worker satisfaction is administered in April and again in October to the same group of workers. If the survey is reliable, and no special program has been introduced between April and October, on average, we would expect satisfaction to remain the same.

The major conceptual difficulty in establishing test-retest reliability is in determining how much time is permissible between the first and second administrations. If too much time elapses, external events might influence responses on the second administration; if too little time passes, the respondents may remember and simply repeat their answers from the first administration.

Equivalence

Equivalence, or alternate-form reliability, refers to the extent to which two assessments measure the same concepts at the same level of difficulty. Suppose that students were given an achievement test before participating in a course and then again two months after completing it. Unless the evaluator is certain that the two tests are of equal difficulty, better performance on the second test could be a result of that test's being easier than the first rather than of improved learning. And, as with test-retest reliability, because this approach requires two administrations, the evaluator must worry about the appropriate interval between them.

As an alternative to establishing equivalence between two forms of the same measure, evaluators sometimes compute a *split-half reliability test*. This requires dividing the measure into two equal halves (or alternate forms) and obtaining the correlation between the two halves. Problems arise if the two halves vary in outcome.

Homogeneity

Homogeneity refers to the extent to which all the items or questions in a measure assess the same skill, characteristic, or quality. Sometimes this type of reliability is referred to as *internal consistency*. The extent of homogeneity is often determined through the calculation of a Cronbach's coefficient alpha, which is basically the average of all the correlations between each item and the total score. For example, suppose that an evaluator has created a questionnaire to find out about patients' satisfaction with Hospital A. An analysis of homogeneity will tell the extent to which all items on the questionnaire focus on satisfaction (rather than some other variable such as knowledge).

Some variables do not have a single dimension. Patient satisfaction, for example, may consist of satisfaction with many elements of the hospital experience: nurses, doctors, financial arrangements, quality of care, quality of surroundings, and so on. If you are unsure of the number of dimensions included in your instrument, you can perform a factor analysis. This statistical procedure identifies relationships among the items or questions in a measure.

Interrater and Intrarater Reliability

Interrater reliability refers to the extent to which two or more individuals agree on a given measurement. Suppose that two individuals are sent to a prenatal care clinic to observe patient waiting times, the appearance of the waiting and examination rooms, and the general atmosphere. If these observers agree perfectly in their ratings of all these items, then interrater reliability is perfect.

Evaluators can enhance interrater reliability by training data collectors thoroughly, providing them with guidelines for recording their observations, monitoring the quality of the data collection over time to ensure that data collectors are not "burning out," and offering data collectors opportunities to discuss any difficult issues or problems they encounter in their work.

Intrarater reliability refers to a single individual's consistency of measurement. Evaluators can also enhance this form of reliability through training, monitoring, and continuous education.

VALIDITY

Validity refers to the degree to which a measure assesses what it purports to measure. For example, a test that asks students to recall information would be considered an invalid measure of their ability to apply information. Similarly, a survey of worker satisfaction cannot be considered valid unless the evaluator can prove that the people who are identified as satisfied based on their responses to the survey think or behave differently than people who are identified as dissatisfied. A measure must be consistent and homogeneous— reliable—to be valid.

Content and Face Validity

Content validity refers to the extent to which a measure thoroughly and appropriately assesses the skills or characteristics it is intended to measure. For example, an evaluator who is interested in developing a measure of quality of life for cancer patients must define *quality of life* and then make sure that items in the measure adequately include all aspects of the definition. Because of the complexity of this task, evaluators will often consult the literature for theories, models, or conceptual frameworks from which to derive the definitions they need. A conceptual model of "quality of life," for instance, consists of the variables included when the concept is discussed in differing kinds of patients, such as those with cancer, those who are depressed, and those who are very old or very young. It is not uncommon for evaluators to make a statement such as the following in establishing content validity: "We used XYZ cognitive theory to select items on knowledge, and we adapted the ABC Role Model Paradigm for questions about social relations."

  Face validity refers to how a measure appears on the surface. Does it seem to ask all the needed questions? Does it use language that is both appropriate and geared to the respondents' reading level to do so? Face validity, unlike content validity, does not rely on established theory for support.

Criterion (Predictive and Concurrent) Validity

Criterion validity is made up of two subcategories: predictive validity and concurrent validity.

  Predictive validity is the extent to which a measure forecasts future performance. A high school entry examination that successfully predicts who will graduate has predictive validity.

  Concurrent validity is demonstrated when two measures produce the same results, or a new measure compares favorably with one that is already considered valid. For example, to establish the concurrent validity of a new aptitude test, the evaluator can administer the new measure as well as a validated measure to the same group of examinees and compare the scores. Alternatively, the evaluator can administer the new test to the examinees and compare the scores with experts' judgment of students' aptitude. A high correlation between the new test and the criterion measure indicates concurrent validity. Establishing concurrent validity is useful when evaluators create a new measure that they believe is better (e.g., shorter, cheaper, fairer) than a previously validated measure.

Construct Validity

Construct validity, which is established experimentally, means that a measure can truly distinguish between people who have certain characteristics and those who do not. For example, an evaluator who claims construct validity for a measure of compassionate nursing care will have to prove in a scientific manner that nurses who do well on the measure are more compassionate than nurses who do poorly. Construct validity is commonly established in at least two ways:

1. The evaluator hypothesizes that the new measure correlates with one or more measures of a similar characteristic (convergent validity) and does not correlate with measures of dissimilar characteristics (discriminant validity). For example, an evaluator who is validating a new quality-of-life measure might hypothesize that it is highly correlated with another quality-of-life instrument, a measure of functioning, and a measure of health status. At the same time, the evaluator might hypothesize that the new measure does not correlate with selected measures of social desirability (individuals' tendency to answer questions to present themselves in a positive light) or measures of hostility.

2. The evaluator hypothesizes that the measure can distinguish one group from the other on some important variable. For example, a measure of compassion should be able to demonstrate that people who are high scorers are compassionate and that people who are low scorers are unfeeling. This requires that the evaluator translate a theory of compassionate behavior into measurable terms, identify people who are compassionate and people who are unfeeling (according to the theory), and prove that the measure consistently and correctly distinguishes between the two groups.

Cultural and Social Validity

Cultural and social validity refers to whether a measure that is developed for one population is meaningful and accurate in another. Constructs such as happiness, self-confidence, pain, depression, and quality of life vary across age, education, and within and across local and national boundaries and cultures. A survey of happiness may produce valid results in a young population but not in an older one or in Country A but not in Country B. If the survey asks questions about job satisfaction, younger people may find the questions relevant, but older retirees will not. Evaluators should conduct pilot tests and consult with users if any doubt exists about a measure's social and cultural validity.

A NOTE ON LANGUAGE: DATA COLLECTION USAGE

The language used to discuss reliability and validity (terms such as *examinees*, *scores*, *scales*, *tests*, and *measures*) comes from test theory, or *psychometrics*. Program evaluators often use the terms *data source*, *measure*, *scale*, *test*, and *instrument* interchangeably. This is sometimes confusing, to say the least, especially because evaluators also talk about *outcome measures* and *outcome indicators* when referring to evaluation study outcomes. The following brief lexicon can be helpful for sorting out data collection terms.

CHECKLIST FOR CREATING A NEW EVALUATION MEASURE

Knowing the types of measures that are available and how to demonstrate their reliability and validity enables the evaluator to get down to the serious business of developing a measure that is tailored to the needs of the investigation or selecting and adapting one that

---

A Guide to Data Collection Terms

- *Data source:* Any source of information for the evaluation. This may include data from questionnaires or tests, literature reviews, and existing databases.
- *Index:* A way of rank ordering things. Scores on an index of function give an indication of where people stand in relation to one another. This term is sometimes used interchangeably with *scale.*
- *Instrument:* A device or strategy used to collect data; instruments include laboratory tests, self-administered questionnaires, and interviews. This term is often used interchangeably with *measure.*
- *Measure:* This term is often used interchangeably with *instrument, test,* and *assessment.* Measures are often the specific devices used in an evaluation such as the 25-item Open City Survey of Student Achievement.
- *Metric:* A way of measuring concepts. If the evaluator uses scores on an achievement test to evaluate an education program, those scores are the metric.
- *Outcome:* The consequences of participating in a program. Outcomes may include improvements in health, education, and welfare.
- *Outcome measure or outcome indicator:* Often used as a synonym for *outcome.*
- *Rating scale:* A graded set of choices. Scales may be nominal (or categorical such as gender, city born in), ordered or ordinal (such as *often, sometimes,* and *never*), or numerical (age, height) and discrete (number of pregnancies, number of arrests for driving drunk). The most used type of rating scale is the Likert scale, with response categories such as *strongly agree, agree, neither agree nor disagree, disagree,* and *strongly disagree.*
- *Scale:* A combination of items or questions that measure the same concept, such as a ten-item scale that measures emotional well-being or a 36-item scale that measures health status.
- *Test:* Achievement test, laboratory test.

---

is already in use. Before you attempt to create a new measure for your evaluation study, you must make sure that you have identified the domain of content (through observation or with the help of experts, research, and theory) and have the expertise, time, and money to complete the task. The following is a checklist of the basic steps you need to take in creating a new measure.

1. **Set boundaries.**
   - *Decide on the type of measure* (e.g., questionnaire, observation).
   - *Determine the amount of needed and available time for administration and scoring* (e.g., a 15-minute interview and ten minutes for summarizing responses).
   - *Select the kinds of reliability and validity information to be collected* (e.g., to establish alternate-form reliability, you must develop two forms; to establish concurrent validity, you will need an already existing instrument).
2. **Define the subject matter or topics that will be covered.** For definitions, consult the literature, experts, or health care consumers. Example 6.1 illustrates how the definitions for an evaluation of prenatal care programs were found in the literature and corroborated by nurses, physicians, and evaluators.

Example 6.1 Defining Terms: The Case of Prenatal Care Programs

Prenatal health care refers to pregnancy-related services provided to a woman between the time of conception and delivery and consists of monitoring the health status of the woman; providing patient information to foster optimal health, good dietary habits, and proper hygiene; and providing appropriate psychological and social support. *Programs* have pre-set, specific purposes and activities for defined populations and groups. *Outcomes of prenatal care programs* include the newborn's gestational age and birth weight and the mother's medical condition and health habits.

These definitions tell the evaluator something like the following: If you want to evaluate prenatal care programs, your measures should include attention to patient education, dietary habits and hygiene, and psychosocial support. If you are interested in outcomes, you will need measures of gestational age and mother's medical condition and health habits. You will also need to decide which medical conditions (e.g., diabetes, hypertension) and health habits (e.g., drinking, smoking) will be the focus of your evaluation.

---

3. **Outline the content.** Suppose that an evaluator is concerned with the outcomes of a particular prenatal care program: the Prenatal Care Access and Utilization Initiative. Assume also that the evaluator's review of the literature and consultation with experts reveal the importance of collecting data on the following variables: still or live birth, birth weight, gestational age, number of prenatal visits, and drug toxicology status of mother and baby. An outline of the contents might look like this:
   a. Baby's birth date
   b. Birth weight
   c. Sex
   d. Gestational age
   e. Whether a drug toxicology screen was performed on baby and results
   f. Whether a drug toxicology screen was performed on mother and result
   g. Number of visits
4. **Select response choices for each question or item.** An *item* on a measure is a question asked of the respondent or a statement to which the respondent is asked to react. Example 6.2 presents a sample item and its response choices.

Example 6.2 Response Choices

Item: What are the test results?   **Choose one**

Choices:
   Normal or negative . . . .   ❐
   Not significant but abnormal . . . .   ❐
   Positive . . . .   ❐
   Equivocal/No data. . . . .   ❐

Selecting response choices for items requires skill and practice. Whenever possible, you should use response choices that others have used effectively. The possibilities of finding appropriate choices are greater when you are collecting demographic information (e.g., age, gender, ethnicity, income, education, where a person lives), for example, than when you are collecting data on the knowledge, attitudes, or behaviors that result from a specific program designed for a particular group of people.

You can find effective item choices in the literature and can obtain many from measures prepared by U.S. Bureau of the Census; the health departments of cities, counties, and states; and other public and private agencies.

5. **Choose rating scales.** You should adapt rating scales from scales that have already been proven in earlier research whenever possible. Like the choices for items, rating scales are available from measures designed by public and private agencies and those described in the literature. Example 6.3 displays an item that uses a simple true-and-false scale.

Example 6.3 Item with a True–False Rating Scale

Please circle the number that best describes whether each of the following statements is true or false for you.

	True	Mostly True	Mostly False	False
I am somewhat ill.	1	2	3	4
I am as healthy as anybody I know.	1	2	3	4
My health is excellent.	1	2	3	4
I have been feeling bad lately.	1	2	3	4

---

6. **Review the measure with experts and potential users.** It is wise to ask other evaluators, subject-matter experts, and potential users (funders, policymakers, other evaluators) and consumers (program and evaluation participants) to review your measure. The following are some important questions to ask them.
7. **Revise the measure based on comments from the reviewers.**
8. **Put the measure in an appropriate format.** For example:
   - Add an ID code, because without such coding you cannot collect data on the same person over time.
   - Add directions for administration and completion.

Questions to Ask of Those Reviewing Your Measure

- **Ask experts.**
  - Is all relevant content covered?
  - Is the content covered in adequate depth?
  - Are all response choices appropriate?
  - Is the measure too long?
- **Ask users and consumers?**
  - Is all relevant content covered?
  - Is the content covered in adequate depth?
  - Do you understand without ambiguity all item choices and scales?
  - Did you have enough time to complete the measure?
  - Did you have enough time to administer the measure?
  - Is the measure too long?

- Add a statement regarding confidentiality (informing the respondent that participants are identifiable by code) or anonymity (informing the respondent that you have no means of identifying participants).
- Add a statement thanking the respondent.
- Give instructions for submitting the completed measure. If it is to be mailed, is an addressed and stamped envelope provided? By what date should the measure be completed?

9. **Review and test the measure before administration.** The importance of pilot-testing a new measure cannot be overemphasized. To conduct a meaningful pilot test, you must use the measure under realistic conditions. This means administering the measure to as many participants as your resources will allow. After they have completed the measure, you need to interview the participants to find out about any problems they might have had in completing the measure. When your study involves interviews, you must test the methods for interviewing as well as the measure itself.

CHECKLIST FOR SELECTING AN ALREADY EXISTING MEASURE

Many instruments and measures are available for use by program evaluators. Good sources for these are the published evaluation reports found in journals. In some cases, whole instruments are published as part of these articles. Even when the measures themselves do not appear, the evaluators usually describe their main data sources and measures in the "methods" sections of their reports, and you can check the references for additional information.

Using an already tested measure has many advantages including saving you the time and other resources needed to develop and validate a completely new instrument. Choosing a measure that has been used elsewhere is not without pitfalls, however. For example, you may have to pay to use an established measure, or you may be required to share your data. You may even have to modify the measure so substantially that its reliability and validity are jeopardized, requiring you to establish them all over again.

The following is a checklist for choosing an already existing measure.

1. **Find out the costs:** Do you have to pay? Share data? Share authorship?
2. **Check the content:** In essence, you must do your own fact and content validity study. Make sure that the questions are the ones you would ask if you were developing the instrument. Check the item choices and rating scales. Will they get you the information you need?
3. **Check the reliability and validity:** Make sure that the types of reliability and validity that have been confirmed are appropriate for your needs. For example, if you are interested in interrater reliability but only internal consistency statistics are provided, the measure may not be the right one for you. If you are interested in a measure's ability to predict but only content validity data is available, think again before adopting the instrument.

You will need to check the context in which the measure has been validated. Are the settings and groups like those in your evaluation? If not, the instrument may not be valid for your purposes. For example, a measure of compliance with counselors' advice in a program to prevent child abuse and neglect that has been tested on teen mothers in Montana may not be applicable to non-teen mothers in Helena, Montana, or to teen mothers in San Francisco, California.

You must also decide whether the measure is sufficiently reliable and valid for use. Reliability and validity are often described as correlations (say, between experts or measures or among items). How high should the correlations be? The fast answer is that the higher, the better, and .90 is best. But the statistic by itself should not be the only or even the most important criterion. A lower correlation may be acceptable if the measure has other properties that are potentially more important. For example, the content may be especially appropriate, or the measure might have been tested on participants who are very much like those in your evaluation.

4. **Check the measure's format:**
   - Will the data collectors be able to score the measure?
   - Does it make sense to use the measure, given your available technology? For example, if the measure requires certain software or expertise, do you have it? Can you afford to get it?
   - Will the participants in the evaluation be willing to complete the measure? Participants sometimes object to spending more than 10–15 minutes on an interview, for example. Also, personal questions and complicated instructions can result in incomplete data.

THE MEASUREMENT CHART: LOGICAL CONNECTIONS

A measurement chart assists the evaluator in the logistics of the evaluation by helping ensure that all variables will have the appropriate coverage. The chart is also useful when the evaluator is writing proposals because it portrays the logical connections among what is being measured, how, for how long, and with whom. When the evaluator is writing reports, the chart provides a summary of some of the important features of the evaluation's data sources. As the sample measurement chart in Table 6.1 illustrates, the information in the chart's columns enables the evaluator to make logical connections among the various segments of data collection. Each column in the chart is explained briefly below it.

Variables: To ensure that all independent and dependent variables are covered, the evaluator uses the table to check the evaluation questions and sampling strategies, including all strata and inclusion and exclusion criteria. For example, suppose that an evaluation asks about the effectiveness of a yearlong combined diet and exercise program in improving the health status and quality of life for people over 75 years of age. Suppose also that it excludes all persons with certain diseases, such as metastatic cancer and heart disease. Assume that the evaluators plan to compare men and women to determine whether any differences exist between them after program participation. The variables needing measurement in such an evaluation would include quality of life, health status (to identify persons with metastatic cancer and heart disease and to assess changes), and demographic characteristics (to determine who is male and who is female).

How measured: For each variable, the measure should be indicated. The measurement chart in Table 6.1 shows that quality of life will be assessed through interviews with patients and observations of how they live, health status will be measured through physical examination, demographic characteristics will be measured through self-administered questionnaires or interviews, and costs will be measured through a review of financial records.

Sample: This column in the measurement chart contains information on the number and characteristics of individuals who will constitute the sample for each measure. For example, the measurement chart in Table 6.1 shows that to measure quality of life, the evaluator will interview all 100 patients (50 men and 50 women) in the experimental group and all 100 patients (50 men and 50 women) in the control group as well as observe a sample of the lifestyles of 50 patients (25 men and 25 women) in each group. Assessment of health status will be based on physical examination of all persons in the experimental and control groups,

Table 6.1 Measurement Chart for an Evaluation of a Health Care Program's Effects on Patient Quality of Life and Health Status

Variables	How Measured	Sample	Timing of Measures	Duration of Measures	Content	Reliability and Validity
Quality of life	Interviews with patients	All 100 patients in the experimental group and all 100 in the control. In each group of 100, 50 men and 50 women	One month before program participation, one month after, and one year after	One-hour interviews; 30 minutes to summarize	Social, emotional, and physical functioning; health beliefs; perceived joy and satisfaction: 35 questions	The Brandyse Functional Assessment (long form) and the University Quality of Living Scale will be adopted. The Brandyse has been validated on 4,000 community-dwelling elderly. Test-retest reliability is .85 and homogeneity for subscales is .90.
	Observations	50 patients in the experimental and 50 in the control groups; 25 men and 25 women in each	One month before program participation and six months after	Half-hour observations; 15 minutes to summarize	Appearance and repair of household; number of visitors; fire and accident safety: ten questions	Interrater reliability will be estimated between at least two observers.
Health status	Physical examination	All persons in experimental and control groups	One month before the program, within one month of completion, and one year later	30 minutes	Emphasis on presence or absence of serious chronic disorders (e.g., metastatic cancer, heart disease): 50 questions	A team of four physicians and nurse practitioners will be trained to administer the physical examinations in a uniform way.
Demographic characteristics	Self-administered questionnaires or interviews	All persons in experimental and control groups	One month before the start of the program	Less than five minutes	Gender, ethnicity, age, education, household income, region of country in which highest level of education was achieved: ten questions	Standard items will be used to collect this data.
Costs	Financial records	All persons receiving care in two clinics, one staffed primarily by physicians and one by nurses	Within one month of completion of the program	About 30 minutes to obtain data and make calculations	Number of staff; hourly wages; number of appointments to each clinic made and kept; number of minutes spent on care	A form will be created, and data collectors will be trained to use it. Periodic quality checks will be made.

and demographic information will be collected on all experimental and control program participants. Data on costs will be collected only for those individuals who use one of the two staffing models.

Timing of measures: The information in this column refers to when each measure is to be administered. For example, the measurement chart in Table 6.1 shows that interviews regarding quality of life and physical examination will be conducted one month before the program, immediately after the program (within one month), and one year after. Observations will be made one month before and six months after. Demographic information will be obtained just once: one month before the start of the program.

Duration of measures: This column of the chart contains information on the amount of time it will take to administer and summarize or score each measure. The measurement chart in Table 6.1 shows that the quality-of-life interviews will take one hour to conduct and 30 minutes to summarize. The observations will take 30 minutes to conduct and 15 minutes to summarize. The physical examinations are expected to take 30 minutes, and collecting data on demographic characteristics will take less than five minutes.

Content: The evaluator should provide a brief description of the content in the measurement chart. For example, if measurement of quality of life is to be based on a particular theory, the evaluator should note the theory's name. If the interview has several sections (e.g., social, emotional, and physical function), the evaluator should mention them. It is important to remember that the chart's purpose is really to serve as a guide to the measurement features of an evaluation. Each one of its sections may require elaboration. For example, for some measures, the evaluator may want to include the number of items in each subscale.

Reliability and validity: If the measures being used are adapted from some other study, the evaluator might describe the relevant types of reliability and validity statistics in this part of the chart. For example, if the quality-of-life measure has been used on older people in another evaluation that showed that higher scorers had higher quality than low scorers, this information might be included. If additional reliability information is to be collected in the current evaluation, that, too, may be reported. A review of medical records to gather information on the number, types, and appropriateness of admissions to the hospital over a one-year period, for example, could require estimations of data collectors' interrater reliability; such information belongs in this section of the chart.

SUMMARY AND TRANSITION TO THE NEXT CHAPTER ON MANAGING EVALUATION DATA AND MANAGING THE EVALUATION

Reliability refers to the consistency of a measure, and *validity* refers to its accuracy. Having reliable and valid measures is essential in an unbiased evaluation. Sometimes the evaluator is required or chooses to create a new measure; at other times, a measure is available that appears to be suitable. Whether creating, adapting, or adopting, the evaluator must critically review the measure to ensure its appropriateness and accuracy for the current study.

A measurement chart is a useful way of showing the relationships among variables, how and when the variables are measured, and the content, reliability, and validity of the measures. Measurement charts are useful tools for evaluators as they plan and report on evaluations.

The next chapter discusses the activities in which the evaluator engages to ensure the proper management of evaluation data to preserve them for analysis. These activities include selecting a database, drafting an analysis plan, creating a codebook, establishing coder reliability, reviewing data collection instruments for incomplete or missing data, entering data into a database, cleaning the data, creating the final data set, sharing and archiving the data set.

EXERCISES: CHAPTER 6

Exercise 1: Reliability and Validity

Directions

Read the following excerpts and determine which concepts of reliability and validity are covered in each.

Excerpt A

The self-administered questionnaire was adapted with minor revisions from the Student Health Risk Questionnaire, which is designed to investigate knowledge, attitudes, behaviors, and various other cognitive variables regarding HIV and AIDS among university students. Four behavior scales measured sexual activity (four questions in each scale) and needle use (five questions); 23 items determined a scale of factual knowledge regarding AIDS. Cognitive variables derived from the health belief model and social learning theory were employed to examine personal beliefs and social norms (12 questions).

Excerpt B

The school's database was reviewed by a single reviewer with expertise in this area; a subset of 35 records was reviewed by a second blinded expert to assess the validity of the review. Rates of agreement for single items ranged from 81% ($\kappa = .77$; $p < .001$) to 100% ($\kappa = 1$; $p < .001$).

Excerpt C

Group A and Group B nurses were given a 22-question quiz that tests evaluation principles derived from the UCLA guidelines. The quizzes were not scored in a blinded manner, but each test was scored twice.

Exercise 2: Reviewing a Data Collection Plan

Directions

Read the following information collection scenario and, acting as an independent reviewer, provide the evaluator with a description of your problems and concerns.

The Department of Sociology is in the process of revising its elective course in research methods. As part of the process, a survey was sent to all faculty who currently teach the methods courses to find out whether and to what extent program evaluation content was covered. Among the expectations was that methods courses would aim to (1) improve students' knowledge of how to design a program evaluation and collect reliable and valid data and (2) prove that all are willing and able to participate in evaluation projects.

The results of the survey revealed little coverage of some important objectives. Many faculty indicated that they would like to include more evaluation content, but they were lacking educational materials and did not have the resources to prepare their own. To rectify this, the Department developed a three-part web-based course. The Center for Evaluation Studies was asked to appraise the effectiveness of the educational materials.

Evaluators from the Center prepared a series of knowledge and skill tests and planned to administer them each year over a five-year period. The evaluators are experts in test construction, and so they decided to omit pilot testing and save time and expense. Their purpose in testing was to measure changes (if any) in students' knowledge of evaluation design and information collection. The evaluators also planned to interview a sample of cooperating students to get an in-depth portrait of their knowledge of program evaluation processes.

SUGGESTED READINGS

Cooper, C. (2023). *An Introduction to Psychometrics and Psychological Assessment*. London and New York: Routledge.

Furr, R.M. (2021). *Psychometrics: An Introduction*. 4th Edition. Los Angeles and London: Sage.

Rust, J., Kosinkski, M., and Stillwell, D. (2021). *Modern Psychometrics: The Science of Psychological Assessment*. 4th Edition. London and New York: Routledge.

ANSWERS TO THE EXERCISES: CHAPTER 6

Exercise 1

Excerpt A: The concept is content validity because the instrument is based on several theoretical constructs (e.g., the health beliefs model and social learning theory).

Excerpt B: The concept is interrater reliability because agreement is correlated between scorers. If we also assume that each expert's ratings are true, then we have concurrent validity; κ (kappa) is a statistic that is used to adjust for agreements that could have arisen by chance alone.

Excerpt C: The concept is test-retest reliability because each test is scored twice.

Exercise 2

This information collection plan has several serious flaws. First, it anticipates collecting data only on student knowledge and skill even though the objectives also encompass attitudes (willingness to participate in evaluation projects). Second, even if the evaluators are expert test constructors, they must pilot test and evaluate the tests to determine their reliability and validity. Finally, the evaluators do not plan to monitor the use of the educational materials. If faculty cannot or will not use these materials, then any results may be spurious. The five-year period planned for testing is, however, probably of sufficient duration to allow the evaluators to observe changes.

CHAPTER 7 | MANAGING EVALUATION DATA AND MANAGING THE EVALUATION

PURPOSE OF CHAPTER 7

The term *data management* refers to what evaluators do with data from the moment it is collected until it is ready to be shared with other evaluators, researchers, program and policy experts, and funders. This chapter discusses how evaluators manage their data by completing nine activities:

1. Selecting a statistical software platform.
2. Drafting an analysis plan that defines and "codes" the variables to be analyzed.
3. Creating a codebook or data dictionary.
4. Ensuring the reliability of the coders.
5. Reviewing the data for completeness and accuracy.
6. Entering data into a database and validating the accuracy of the entry.
7. Cleaning the data.
8. Creating the final data set for analysis.
9. Storing and archiving the data.

A READER'S GUIDE TO CHAPTER 7

What Is Data Management?
Selecting a Statistical Software Platform
Drafting an Analysis Plan
Creating a Codebook or Data Dictionary
    Ensuring Reliable Coding
    Measuring Agreement: The Kappa
Entering the Data
Searching for Missing Data
    What to Do When Participants Omit Information
Cleaning the Data
    Outliers
    When Data Needs Recoding
Creating the Final Database for Analysis
Storing and Archiving the Database

DOI: 10.4324/9781032635071-7

WHAT IS DATA MANAGEMENT?

The term *data management* refers to what evaluators do with data from the moment it is collected until it is ready to be shared with other evaluators, researchers, program developers and participants, policy experts, and funders.

Evaluation data management activities include at least nine activities:

1. Selecting a statistical software platform.
2. Drafting an analysis plan that defines and "codes" the variables to be analyzed.
3. Creating a codebook or data dictionary (an "operations" manual).
4. Ensuring the reliability of the coders.
5. Reviewing the data for completeness and accuracy.
6. Entering data into a database and validating the accuracy of the entry.
7. Cleaning the data.
8. Creating the final data set for analysis.
9. Storing and archiving the data.

SELECTING A STATISTICAL SOFTWARE PLATFORM

An unbiased evaluation is dependent upon the validity of the data it collects and analyzes. It is therefore conditional upon accurate data entry and a carefully constructed database. When evaluators talk about data entry, they mean the process of digitizing data by entering it into a database for organization and management purposes. Evaluators can either select their own database entry and management systems or they may rely on those provided by the institutions for which they work. All major statistical programs, such as SAS or SPSS, offer the evaluation team comprehensive computing and management systems.

The complexity and importance of data management are sometimes overlooked, even though evaluators estimate that data management activities take up between 20% and 50% of the time typically allocated for the analytic process. As you plan your own evaluation, it is important that you be realistic about the amount of time you will need for data management, and that you make sure you have sufficient resources (skills, staff, time, money) to do the job. The principles that underlie good data management apply to qualitative data as well as to statistical information.

DRAFTING AN ANALYSIS PLAN

An analysis plan contains a description and explanation of the statistical and other analytic methods that the evaluator plans to use with the data that has been collected to answer each evaluation question or test each hypothesis.

Suppose that you are the evaluator of a health education program designed to reduce risks for harmful drinking among adults. The program consists of three main components: (a) the Alcohol-Related Problems Screen (ARPS), a measure to determine drinking classification (harmful or not harmful); (b) a report describing the reasons for an individual's classification (such as "A person who drinks four or more drinks at one sitting two or three times a week or more is a harmful drinker"); and (c) educational materials (a booklet and a list of related websites) to help people cut their drinking down to a healthier level.

Example 7.1 shows portions of a simple plan for analyzing the data to answer two of this study's evaluation questions.

Example 7.1 Portion of an Analysis Plan for an Evaluation of a Program to Reduce Harmful Drinking in Adults

Evaluation Question 1

Question: How do men and women compare in terms of numbers of harmful drinkers?

Hypothesis: More men than women will be harmful drinkers.

Independent variable: Gender.

Data source: Survey questionnaire (Are you male or female?).

Dependent variable: Drinking status (harmful or not harmful).

Data source: The Alcohol-Related Problems Screen.

Planned analysis: Chi-square to test for differences between numbers of men and women who are or are not harmful drinkers, according to their scores on the Alcohol-Related Problems Screen.

Evaluation Question 2

Question: How do men and women compare in their risks for harmful drinking as defined by scores on the Alcohol-Related Problems Screen?

Independent variable: Gender.

Data source: Survey questionnaire (Are you male or female?).

Dependent variable: Risks for harmful drinking.

Data source: The Alcohol-Related Problems Screen. (Higher scores mean greater risks. Scores are continuous and range from 1 to 50.)

Planned analysis: t-test to test for differences in average scores obtained by men and by women.

The evaluation questions and hypothesis contain the independent and dependent or outcome variables. Each variable has a source of data (survey questionnaire, the Alcohol-Related Problems Screen). The data has certain characteristics. In Example 7.1, it is categorical (male or female; harmful or not harmful) or continuous (a score of 1 to 5). You need to understand the characteristics of the data to choose an appropriate statistical technique. Categorical data lends itself to analytic methods (such as chi-square) that differ from those used with continuous data (such as a t-test).

Regardless of how well you plan your analysis, the realities of sampling and data collection may force you to modify your plan. Suppose, for example, that you review preliminary data from the Alcohol-Related Problems Screen (Evaluation Question 2 in Example 7.1). Based on the results of your review, you decide that in addition to testing for differences in average scores, you also want to compare the number of men and women who attain scores of 25 or higher with the number who obtain scores of 24 or lower. You would then have to modify your original analysis plan to include a chi-square test (to compare proportions or numbers). In general, evaluators can count on having to make modifications to their original analysis plans, especially in large studies that collect a great deal of data.

CREATING A CODEBOOK OR DATA DICTIONARY

Codes are units that the evaluator uses to "speak" to the statistical or qualitative software. Suppose that in your evaluation of a program to reduce harmful drinking, 1,000 men and women complete the Alcohol-Related Problems Screen. This survey of alcohol use asks respondents how much and how often they drink. To determine how many men report drinking four drinks at one sitting two or three times a week, for example, you will have to communicate with the statistical software program and "tell" it which variables to look for (e.g., gender and quantity and frequency of alcohol use). Software programs read variables through codes. Example 7.2 displays two items from the Alcohol-Related Problems Screen.

Example 7.2 Excerpts from a Screening Measure to Detect Harmful Drinking

1. Are you male or female? **[GNDR]**

    Male $\square_0$

    Female $\square_1$

    Prefer not to say $\square_2$

8. How often in the past 12 months have you had four or more drinks of alcohol at one sitting? **[QFDRINK]**

    Choose one answer.

    Daily or almost daily $\square_1$

    Four or five times a week $\square_2$

    Two or three times a week $\square_3$

    Two to four times a month $\square_4$

    One time a month or less $\square_5$

    Never $\square_0$

In Example 7.2, the codes are the numbers to the right of the response boxes. You use a statistical program to tell you how many people who answered "1" to question 1 also answered "4" to question 8. To do this, you must tell the program the names of the variables (Question 1 = GNDR and Question 8 = QFDRINK) and their values (0 = male and 1 = female; 1 = daily or almost daily to 0 = never). Many statistical programs also require that you tell the computer where in the data line to find the variables. (See the section "Entering the Data," later in this chapter.) The "words" in brackets in Example 7.2 (GNDR and QFDRINK) correspond to the variables represented by each question.

The evaluator must create a *codebook* or *data dictionary* that contains descriptions of all the questions, codes, and variables associated with a survey. Example 7.3 displays portions of a typical codebook.

Example 7.3 Portions of a Codebook

Variable Name	Variable Label	Values: Labels and Codes
PROJID	Project code	7-digit ID
AGE	Age	Date of birth: Month/day/year
GNDR	GNDR	Gender of respondent: 0 = male; 1 = female.; 3 = prefer not to say Leave blank if missing
CNTRY	Country born in	Country person is born in: 01 = Argentina; 02 = Bolivia; 03 = Chile; 04 = Colombia; 05 = Cuba; 06 = Ecuador; 07 = El Salvador; 08 = Guatemala; 09 = Honduras; 10 = Mexico; 11 = Nicaragua; 12 = Peru; 13 = Puerto Rico Leave blank if no data
GUILT	Feels guilty or sorry	1 = daily or almost daily; 2 = at least once a week, but less than daily; 3 = at least once a month, but less than weekly; 4 = less than once a month; 0 = never Leave blank if no data
DRIVE	Drinks and drives	1 = 20 or more days; 2 = 10–19 days; 3 = 6–9 days; 4 = 3–5 days; 5 = 1–2 days; 0 = never Leave blank if no data

As this example illustrates, each variable is broken down into discrete units, called *values*, that correspond to the codes for that variable. For instance, participants' feeling guilty or sorry for something they did because of alcohol use has five values: 1 = daily or almost daily; 2 = at least once a week but less than daily; 3 = at least once a month but less than weekly; 4 = less than once a month; 0 = never. The codes are thus 0, 1, 2, 3, and 4. The codebook also notes that if no information is available, nothing is filled in.

The evaluator should assign missing data a code or value that is not numeric, because many statistical programs will treat all codes as data that needs to be analyzed. Suppose that you are conducting a survey of teens, and one participant neglects to include his or her age on a questionnaire; if you code that missing information as 99, the statistical program will likely assume that the respondent is 99 years old.

There are several ways to code missing data, including using a period (.) or inserting a blank space. Some software programs allow users to select several codes for missing data, such as ".a" for missing, ".b" for "don't know," and ".c" for "not applicable." It is a good idea to distinguish among these three concepts. If a person in an evaluation of harmful drinking does not drink, for instance, then all variables pertaining to the quantity and frequency of that person's drinking should be coded as "not applicable," given that the data is not actually "missing." When you have selected the software you will use in your evaluation, check the manual to see which coding system is appropriate and to determine what will work best for your analysis.

Although statistical software programs vary in the terminology they use, many (but by no means all) require that variable labels appear in all capital letters (PQOL or EDUC) and do not permit the use of special characters (such as commas and semicolons) in these labels. Some programs limit the number of characters for variable labels to about eight. Variable labels should be based on the actual names of the variables (e.g., the variable name "perceived quality of life" is given the variable label PQOL). To understand the data, the software needs to know the name of each variable, the variable's label, and the variable's values and their labels. For the variable named "community," for example, the software needs to know that its label is COMM and that its values are 1 = urban and 2 = rural. (Note that although the statistical program you use may employ slightly different terms for all these concepts, the ideas will be the same.)

Ensuring Reliable Coding

To ensure reliable data in a small evaluation—say, with just one person doing the coding—the evaluator should recode all or a sample of the data to check for consistency. The second coding should take place about a week after the first coding. This is enough time for the coder to forget the first set of codes so that he or she does not just automatically reproduce them. After the data is coded a second time, the evaluator should compare the two sets of codes for agreement. If there are disagreements, the evaluator may resolve them by calling in a second person to arbitrate.

In a large evaluation, a second person should independently code a sample of the data. To assure reliability between coders, the evaluator must provide the coders with formal training and make sure they have access to the definitions of all terms.

Despite the evaluator's best efforts at setting up a high-quality codebook and data management system, the coders may not always agree with one another. To find out the extent of agreement between coders—intercoder or interrater reliability—the evaluator can calculate a statistic called *kappa*, which measures how much better than chance the agreement between a given pair of coders is. The following subsection explains the principle behind the kappa statistic.

Measuring Agreement: The Kappa

Suppose that two evaluators are each asked to review 100 interviews with single working mothers of two or more children. These mothers have just completed a month-long program, and the interviews are about their health-related quality of life. The reviewers are to study the transcripts of the interviews to find how many of the participants mention doing regular exercise during the discussion. The reviewers are asked to code 0, for "no," if a participant does not mention regular exercise at least once, and 1, for "yes," if she does mention regular exercise. Here are the reviewers' codes:

Reviewer 2	Reviewer 1		
	No	**Yes**	
No	20^C	15	35^B
Yes	10	55^D	65
	30^A	70	

Reviewer 1 says that 30 (A) of the 100 interviews do not contain reference to regular exercise, whereas Reviewer 2 says that 35 (B) do not. The two reviewers agree that 20 (C) interviews do not include mention of exercise.

What is the best way to describe the extent of agreement between these reviewers? The figure of 20 out of 100, or 20% (C), is probably too low, because the reviewers also agree that 55% (D) of the interviews include mention of exercise. The total agreement 55% + 20% is an overestimate, because with only two categories (yes and no), some agreement may occur by chance. This is shown in the following formula, in which O is the observed agreement and C is the chance agreement.

Measuring Agreement Between Two Coders: The Kappa (κ) Statistic

$$k = \frac{O - C}{1 - C},$$

where $O - C$ = agreement beyond chance and $1 - C$ = agreement possible beyond chance. Here is how this formula works with the above example.

1. Calculate how many interviews the reviewers may agree by chance *do not* include mention of exercise. One does this by multiplying the number of no's and dividing by 100, because there are 100 interviews: $(30 \times 35)/100 = 10.5$.
2. Calculate how many interviews the reviewers may agree by chance *do* include mention of exercise by multiplying the number of interviews that each reviewer found to include mention. One does this by multiplying the number of yeses and dividing by 100: $(70 \times 65)/100 = 45.5$.
3. Add the two numbers obtained in steps 1 and 2 and divide by 100 to get a proportion for *chance agreement*: $(10.5 + 45.5)/100 = 0.56$.

The *observed agreement* is 20% + 55% = 75%, or 0.75. Therefore, the agreement beyond chance is 0.75 − 0.56 = 0.19: the numerator.

The *agreement possible beyond chance* is 100% minus the chance agreement of 56%, or 1 − 0.56 = 0.44: the denominator.

$$k = \frac{0.19}{0.44} \quad k = 0.43$$

What is a "high" kappa? Some experts have attached the following qualitative terms to kappas: 0.0–0.2 = slight, 0.2–0.4 = fair, 0.4–0.6 = moderate, 0.6–0.8 = substantial, and 0.8–0.10 = almost perfect.

How can an evaluator achieve substantial or almost perfect agreement—reliability—among reviewers? By making certain that all reviewers collect and record data on the same topics and that they agree in advance on what each important variable means. The "fair" kappa of 0.43 obtained by the reviewers in the example above may be due to differences between the reviewers' and the evaluator's definitions, the evaluator's poor training of the reviewers in the use of the definitions, and/or mistakes in coding.

ENTERING THE DATA

Data entry is the process of getting evaluation information from surveys, interviews, observations, records, and other measures into a database. Entry usually takes one of three forms. In the first form, the evaluator hand enters the data into a database management or spreadsheet program. In the second form, the evaluator scans the data (such as a page of a completed survey) using a combined OCR/OMR system (optical character recognition and optical mark recognition). The OCR/OMR system "reads" the data and processes it electronically. In the third form of data entry, data is automatically entered into a database as the evaluator or participant completes data collection. Most survey software packages provide this function.

Each data entry, database management, and statistical program has its own conventions and terminology. Some programs refer to entering data as setting up a "record" for each evaluation participant. The record consists of the participant's unique ID (identification code) and the participant's "observations" (response choices, scores, comments, and so on). Other programs consider the unit of analysis (such as the individual participant) as the observation, and the data collected on each observation is referred to as "variables" or "fields."

Example 7.4 shows a simple data set for six people.

Example 7.4 Data on Six People

RESPID	GNDR	MARRIED	CHILDREN	GUILTY	REPORT
1	1	3	2	1	1
2	2	4	1	3	2
3	2	3	2	3	2
4	1	3	2	1	2
5	3	1	1	1	2
6	1	3	1	3	1

In this example, the table is organized so that, except for the first column, the participants' identification (RESPID) numbers constitute the rows and the data on the participants is the columns. That is, person 2's data is 2, 4, 1, 3, and 2. Many statistical programs require the user to tell the computer where on the data line a variable is located. For instance, in Example 7.6 the person's gender is called GNDR, and data on gender can be found in column 2. Feeling guilty because of drinking is called GUILT, and the data for this variable can be found in column 5.

Database management programs, statistical programs, and online surveys with automatic data entry can facilitate the accuracy of data entry when they are programmed to allow the entry of only "legal" codes. For instance, if the codes should be entered as 001, 002, and so on, up to 010, the user can write rules so that an entry of 01 or 10 is not permitted—that is, if anyone tries to enter 01 or 10, the program will respond with an error message. With minimal programming, such software can also check each entry to ensure that it is consistent with previously entered data and that skip patterns in the questionnaire are respected. That is, the program can make sure that the fields for questions that are to be skipped by some participants are coded as skips and not as missing data. Designing a data entry protocol requires skill and time. The evaluator should never regard any such protocol as error-free until it has been tested and retested in the field.

SEARCHING FOR MISSING DATA

The evaluator should review the first completed data collection instruments as soon as they are available. In any study using self-administered surveys (which includes many evaluations), the evaluator can expect to find some survey questions unanswered. Participants may not answer questions for many reasons. For example, they may not want to answer some questions, or they may not understand what they are being asked to do. Some participants may not understand the directions for completing a survey because the questionnaire requires them to read too much or is composed at a level beyond their reading capabilities.

Participants in print surveys may be unsure about what methods they should use in responding (e.g., whether they should fill in boxes completely or mark them with checks, whether they should circle the correct answers). They may find that questions are presented in a format that is difficult to use, such as the one in Example 7.5.

Example 7.5 A Question That May Be Confusing

Please cross out the choice that best describes you. An example of a cross out is:

~~Lots of times~~

Please answer ALL questions.

32. How often over the past year have you told others that you would hurt them?	~~Never~~	Sometimes	Lots of times	Almost every day
33. How often over the past year have you slapped, punched, or hit someone before they hit you?	Never	Sometimes	Lots of times	Almost every day
34. How often over the past year have you slapped, hit, or punched someone after they hit you?	Never	Sometimes	Lots of times	Almost every day
35. How often over the past year have you beaten up someone?	Never	Sometimes	Lots of times	Almost every day
36. How often over the past year have you attacked or stabbed someone with a knife?	Never	Sometimes	Lots of times	Almost every day

In Example 7.5, the participant has answered just one question even though he or she was asked to answer all the questions. What do the unanswered items mean? Has the participant declined to answer the questions because the behaviors described are too personal or too offensive? Would the response rate have improved if the evaluator had added a choice like "prefer not to answer"? In fact, the format of the question may have been the problem.

The evaluator who designed the question in Example 7.5 probably used this tabular format to save space and to avoid repeating the response choices over and over. Participants may find such a format confusing because it is different from the typical multiple-choice format.

Confusing question formats lead to missing data because participants do not know how to answer the questions and leave them blank. The evaluator may overcome some of the problems that cause participants to misunderstand survey questions by conducting extensive cognitive pretests and pilot tests. *Cognitive pretests* are interviews with potential participants in which they are asked to interpret each question and response choice on a survey. *Pilot tests* are tests of the survey questions in the actual evaluation setting. These two activities will tell evaluators if a particular question format is unusable or some questions do not make sense, enabling problems to be addressed before data collection begins.

What to Do When Participants Omit Information

Say that you mail 100 25-item questionnaires and get 95 back. You proudly announce that you have a 95% response rate for your questionnaire. Then, on closer examination, you discover that half the participants did not answer question 5, and that each of the remaining 24 survey questions also has missing data. With all that missing information, you cannot really claim to have a 95% response rate for all questions.

What should an evaluator do about missing responses? In some program evaluations, it may be possible to go back to the participants and ask them to answer the questions they left unanswered. In small studies where the participants are known (such as within one school or clinic), the evaluator may be able to contact the participants easily. But in most surveys, collecting information a second time is usually impractical, if not impossible. Some evaluations, for example, use anonymous data collection methods, and so the evaluators do not even know who the participants are. In an institutional setting, the evaluator may have to go back to the ethics board to get permission to contact the participants a second time—a process that takes time and may delay completion of the evaluation, and so is rarely done.

In online data collection, surveys can be programmed so that the respondent must answer one question before proceeding to the next. This approach can help to minimize the amount of missing data. However, evaluation participants may find this restriction frustrating and give up on the survey. Some evaluators believe that forcing participants to answer every question is coercive and unethical. In their view, a program that forces respondents to answer a question, even if they prefer not to, violates the ethics principle of autonomy, or respect for individuals. Moreover, using this approach may result in unreliable information, as some people may enter meaningless answers to some questions just to be able to move on in the survey.

Evaluators often use a statistical method called *weighting* to make up for nonresponse. Suppose that you expect 50% of men and 50% of women in a sample to complete a survey, but only 40% of men do. In such a case, you can weight the men's returns so that they are equivalent to 50%. There are several strategies for weighting, among them logistic regression analysis. In this method, the existence or nonexistence of a response is considered a dichotomous dependent variable and other variables are used to predict it. Dichotomous variables are divided into two components. For instance, if the variable "age" is dichotomous, then it is divided into two parts, such as 65 and older and 64 and younger. Scores can be dichotomized: on a ten-item test, scores of 5 or more versus scores of 4 and under.

Suppose that you have information on age and gender, *and* you can predict whether a person responded using these two variables—that is, your participants and nonparticipants differ on these characteristics. Logistic regression provides you with an estimate of the probability that a given respondent's data will be missing. The probabilities are assigned as weights for all cases. Cases that have missing data are given higher weights. All statistical software programs include mechanisms for weighting responses.

Another commonly used statistical method to account for missing data is the last observation *carried forward* (LOCF). LOCF uses the last value observed before the participant left, regardless of when the dropout occurred. LOCF makes the probably unrealistic assumption that participants who drop out would continue responding precisely as they did at the time of drop out. Because of this assumption, LOCF is losing favor. Newer methods use statistical models in which each participant is fitted with her own regression line over time, so that when a participant drops out, her curve is projected to the end of the study, rather than simply holding at whatever the last value was, as in LOCF.

Missing data is sometime handled by filling in a "reasonable" value such as an average score for each participant who did respond. Suppose Participant A did not answer a survey question about his annual household income. To fill in the blank with a reasonable value, the researcher can compute the average of all participants' responses to the question and use the average as the value for Participant A. The reasoning behind this approach is that Participant A is unlikely to deviate substantially from the average person in the study. This approach probably works, however, only if just a few respondents leave out a particular question, and if the researchers have no reason to think that any given respondent is different, on average, from the others.

It has become standard practice in randomized controlled trials to use an *intention-to-treat analysis* (ITT) to handle the drop-out problem. With this type of analysis, all participants are included in the study group to which they were allocated, whether they received (or completed) the program given to that group. Analyze as randomized! ITT's critics assert that its use may underestimate the full effects of a program because some people are included who did not receive the intended program. As an alternative to ITT, some evaluators use *per protocol analysis* in which only participants who complete the entire program are included in the analysis. Per protocol analysis critics argue that this technique may result in an overestimation of effectiveness.

Loss of study information from attrition or refusal or inability to complete data collection can be a very serious problem. Statistical fixes are complex and controversial, and most evaluators try to avoid the problem to begin with.

Experienced evaluators avoid missing data by being realistic about the study's inclusion and exclusion criteria, training and monitoring project staff to recruit and work with participants effectively, reimbursing participants for spending their time to complete study activities, providing participants with readable updates on individual and study progress, ensuring informed consent, and keeping all information confidential.

CLEANING THE DATA

Once the data is entered, it needs to be cleaned. When a data set is clean, anyone who uses it will get the same results when running analyses. Data becomes "dirty" for several reasons including miscoding and incorrect data entry. To avoid dirty data, the evaluator must make sure that coders and data entry personnel are experienced, well trained, and properly supervised. One way of checking the data is to compare variable values against preset maximum and minimum levels. If, for example, someone enters 50 when the maximum is 5, an error has clearly occurred. The evaluator can also minimize errors by making sure that the coding scheme distinguishes truly missing data (no response or no data) from responses of "don't know" or "not applicable."

The evaluator should run frequencies or descriptive statistics (such as tabulations of the responses to a survey's question) on the data as soon as about 10% of the responses are in, and then run them again and again until data collection is running smoothly. If the data set is relatively small, the evaluator can visually scan the frequencies for errors. For large databases with data from many measures and variables and from surveys with skip patterns and open-ended text responses, a systematic computerized check may be required. All leading statistical programs contain cleaning specifications that can be used during data entry and later as a separate data cleaning process.

Several other problems may require the evaluator to clean up the data. These include information collection measures that have not been completed at all, others that have been only partially completed, and still others that contain data that are very different from those of the average evaluation participant.

Outliers

Outliers are data or observations that appear inconsistent with the rest of the data set. They may be detected by a statistical program's built-in checks, or the evaluator may discover them by running frequencies and other descriptive statistics and checking the results against acceptable values. For instance, suppose that you survey 50 people to find out if they like a particular movie. You review the returns and find that 48 participants assigned ratings of 2, 3, and 4 on a scale of 1 (*hated it*) to 5 (*loved it*). One respondent is consistently negative and assigns ratings of 1 to all 75 questions about the movie. Another respondent assigns ratings of 5 to all 75 questions. These two people may be outliers—the question is what to do about them.

Some evaluators simply discard outliers from their data analyses. Each evaluator must decide on a case-by-case basis what to do with data that clearly deviates from the norm. Such decisions should be made with caution: When you discard seemingly deviant data, you may also be tossing out important information. Methods of detecting outliers include regression analysis and formal tests that assume that variables are normally distributed. (See Chapter 8 for a discussion of the normal distribution.)

When Data Needs Recoding

Data management will continue until the evaluation's last analysis is performed. For example, as time goes on, you may want to add additional people to the evaluation, or you may want to consider studying additional variables. These activities will require coding, data entry, and data cleaning. You may need to recode the data you have collected, as illustrated in Example 7.6.

Example 7.6 Recoding Data

Example 1: A program is initiated to encourage 15 communities to participate in a collaborative community evaluation. About one-third of the community's representatives think collaboration is a waste of time. After the two-day program is completed, the evaluators interview the participants to find out whether their attitudes have changed. The evaluators hypothesize that the older participants are more interested in collaboration than the younger ones. They have data on each person's birth date, and preliminary analysis reveals that the participants' ages range from 26 to 71. The median age of the sample is 42. The evaluators decide to compare the attitudes of older and younger people. They recode the data to make two age categories: 42 and younger and 43 and older.

Example 2: The evaluators of an intervention to improve family function adopt a standardized measure of family stability. The measure has ten items, each rated on a scale of 1 to 5. The evaluators discover that seven of the items are worded so that a score of 1 is high and a score of 5 is low. On the other three items, a score of 5 is high and a score of 1 is low. Because the evaluators want a total score of family stability, they must recode the three reverse-worded questions so that a 1 is scored as if it were a 5, a 2 as if it were a 4, and so on. If they do not recode the data, the items will not have a common direction, and the evaluators will be unable to sum them to get a score.

CREATING THE FINAL DATABASE FOR ANALYSIS

Once data analysis begins, the evaluator may alter the characteristics of some of the variables so that continuous variables are dichotomized, and new categories and derived variables are created. Example 7.7 shows how this works.

Example 7.7 On the Way to an Analytic Data Set

Continuous Variables Are Dichotomized

1. Scores on the DRINK measure range from 1 to 100. For the analysis, the evaluators compare persons with scores of 25 and less with those who achieved 26 or more.
2. The Alcohol-Related Problems Screen (ARPS) asks participants to complete this question:

During the past 12 months, how often did you have six or more drinks of alcohol at one sitting?

	Please check one.
Daily or almost daily.....................................	❏
Four or five times a week..............................	❏
Two or three times a week	❏
Two to four times a month	❏
One time a month or less...............................	❏

Because the evaluators are concerned with comparing people who drink in excess of recommended limits with those who do not, they dichotomize the answers to this question by comparing the proportion of participants who answer "never" to those who give any other response.

New Categories Are Created

The ARPS lists several medications and asks participants to check off the ones they are taking. The evaluators decide to group the specific medications into categories, such as antidepressants, antihypertensives, and so on.

Derived Variables Are Produced

The evaluators create a variable called "drink years" by multiplying years of drinking times number of drinks per day.

STORING AND ARCHIVING THE DATABASE

The evaluator must be sure to create backup copies of the database and the analytic data set, and record in the codebook all changes that were made to the database or data set. Once the evaluator is confident that the data is clean and that all changes to the database are final and documented, the analysis can begin.

The file format you choose for the data really matters to someone else's ability to access and use the database in the future. Technology continually changes and all contemporary hardware and software becomes unusable or inaccessible every few years. Take the time to consider how your data will be read if the software used to produce it becomes unavailable. Although any file format you choose today may become unreadable in the future, some formats are more likely to be readable than others. Data management specialists suggest that the formats meet these criteria: The formats are not proprietary; they are open with documented standards; and they use standard character encodings such as ASCII and UTF-8. Text should be TXT, HTML, SML, or PDF/A. Databases should be preserved as XML or CSV files.

SUMMARY AND TRANSITION TO THE NEXT CHAPTER ON ANALYZING EVALUATION DATA

This chapter discussed the activities that evaluators engage in to ensure the proper management of evaluation data so that the data is ready for analysis and sharing. These activities include selecting a database platform, drafting an analysis plan, creating a codebook, establishing coder reliability, reviewing collected data for incomplete or missing responses, entering data into a database, cleaning the data, creating the final data set, and archiving, securing, and readying the data for sharing.

The next chapter focuses on data analysis methods that are particularly useful in program evaluations. It describes how the evaluator should go about determining the characteristics of the data that describe or measure each main variable and which subsequently determine which analytic strategy is appropriate. The next chapter also discusses how to establish practical as well as statistical meaning by confidence intervals and other techniques. Special statistical tests involving odds and risks are discussed because of their importance in evaluation studies. In addition, the chapter discusses the analysis of qualitative data and meta-analysis.

EXERCISES: CHAPTER 7

Exercise 1

Directions

Interpret the codes for the following question asked on a telephone interview. The codes are in brackets.

[T_9] How much of the time during the PAST 4 WEEKS have you felt calm and peaceful? Would you say all of the time, most of the time, some of the time, a little of the time, or none of the time?

All of the time	❏	[100]
Most of the time	❏	[75]
Some of the time	❏	[50]
A little of the time	❏	[25]
None of the time	❏	[0]
DON'T KNOW	❏	[8]
REFUSED	❏	[9]

Exercise 2

Directions

Assign codes to this set of questions asked during the same telephone interview as in Exercise 1.

My illness has strengthened my faith. Would you say this statement is very much, quite a bit, somewhat, a little bit, or not at all true?

Very much	❏
Quite a bit	❏
Somewhat	❏
A little bit	❏
Not at all	❏
DON'T KNOW	❏
REFUSED	❏

How much time during the LAST 4 WEEKS have you wished that you could change your mind about the kind of treatment you chose for prostate cancer? Would you say all of the time, most of the time, a good bit of the time, some of the time, a little of the time, or none of the time?

All of the time	❏
Most of the time	❏
A good bit of the time	❏
Some of the time	❏
A little of the time	❏
None of the time	❏
DON'T KNOW	❏
REFUSED	❏

SUGGESTED READING

Briney, K. (2015). *Data management for researchers: Organize, maintain and share your data for research success*. Pellagic Publishing

Corti, L., Van den Eynden, V, Bishop, L., & Woolard, M. (2019). *Managing and sharing research data: A guide to good practice*. Second Edition. Sage.

Kanza, S. & Knight, N.J. (2022). Behind every great research project is great data management. *BMC Research Notes*, *15*(20). https://doi.org/10.1186/s13104-022-05908-5.

Krishnankutty, B., Bellary, S., Kumar, N.B.R., & Moodahadu, L.S. (2012). Data management in clinical research: An overview. *Indian Journal of Pharmacology*, *44*(2): 168–172.

Suggested Websites

What Is Research Data Management
https://datamanagement.hms.harvard.edu/about/what-research-data-management

Research Data Management and Sharing
www.coursera.org/learn/data-management

What Is Data Management, and Why Is it Important?
https://guides.library.cmu.edu/c.php?g=1136565&p=8295133

ANSWERS TO THE EXERCISES: CHAPTER 7

Exercise 1

- The "T" stands for "telephone" and the "_9" stands for the "ninth question."
- "All of the time" is coded 100; "most of the time," 75; "some of the time," 50; "a little of the time," 25; "none of the time," 0; "don't know," 8; and "refused," 9.
- The codes of 100, 75, 50, and 25 allow the data analyst to compute a "score."

Exercise 2

[T_1] My illness has strengthened my faith. Would you say this statement is very much, quite a bit, somewhat, a little bit, or not at all true.

Very much_	(4)
Quite a bit_	(3)
Somewhat_	(2)
A little bit_	(1)
Not at all_	(0)
DON'T KNOW_	(8)
REFUSED_	(9)

2 (a) [T_2] How much of the time during the LAST 4 WEEKS have you wished that you could change your mind about the kind of treatment you chose for prostate cancer? Would you say all of the time, most of the time, a good bit of the time, some of the time, a little of the time, or none of the time?

Very much_	(4)
Quite a bit_	(3)
Somewhat_	(2)
A little bit_	(1)
Not at all_	(0)
DON'T KNOW_	(8)
REFUSED_	(9)

Note that because 8 and 9 are used as codes in the first question, these codes are repeated in the answers to the second. It is always a good idea to keep codes consistent in all evaluation data collection measures.

CHAPTER 8 | ANALYZING EVALUATION DATA

PURPOSE OF CHAPTER 8

Program evaluators use statistical and qualitative methods to analyze data and answer questions about program effectiveness, quality, and value. This chapter explains why data analysis depends as much on the characteristics of the evaluation's questions and the quality of its data as it does on the evaluator's skills in doing the analysis. The chapter also discusses the logic that evaluators use to plan data analysis.

Program evaluators use statistical methods to analyze data, and so this chapter covers hypothesis testing, confidence intervals, odds and risks, and meta-analyses. Finally, because evaluators may use qualitative as well as statistical methods, the chapter includes a discussion of one commonly used qualitative method: content analysis.

A READER'S GUIDE TO CHAPTER 8

DOI: 10.4324/9781032635071-8

Summary and Transition to the Next Chapter on Evaluation Reports
Exercises: Chapter 8
Suggested Reading
  Suggested Websites
Answers to Exercises: Chapter 8

START WITH THE EVALUATION QUESTIONS AND EVIDENCE OF EFFECTIVENESS, QUALITY, AND VALUE

Planning for data begins with a review of the evaluation questions and hypothesis and evidence of effectiveness, quality, and value. Planning and requires the answers to three questions:

1. What are the characteristics of the data collected for each independent and each dependent variable? Quantitative data may be characterized as categorical (male, female), ordinal (high, medium, low), or numerical (a score of 30 out of 100 possible points). Qualitative data is often summarized in terms of the themes that emerge repeatedly from participants' comments and evaluators' observations.
2. Which statistical or qualitative methods are appropriate for answering the evaluation questions and providing evidence, given the data's characteristics?
3. If a statistical method is appropriate, do the evaluation's data meet all its assumptions? For example, is the data "normally distributed"?

CATEGORICAL, ORDINAL, AND NUMERICAL DATA

The first step in selecting an analytic method is to identify the characteristics of the data collected for each independent and each dependent variable specified in the evaluation question. Independent variables are used to explain or predict a program's outcomes (the dependent variables). Typical independent variables in program evaluations include group membership (experimental and control program) and demographic characteristics such as age, income, and education. Typical dependent variables in evaluations include knowledge, attitudes and social, educational, and health behavior. Evaluation data takes three forms: *categorical*, *ordinal*, and *numerical*.

Categorical Data

Categorical data comes from asking for information that fits into categories. For example:

What is the student's gender?	
Male	❐
Female	❐
Check the student's favorite type of reading.	
Fiction	❐
History	❐
Mystery	❐
Biography	❐

Both questions require the participant to select the category (male, female) into which the response to the questions—the data—fits. When categorical data takes on one of two values (e.g., male or female; yes or no), they are termed *dichotomous* (as in "divided in two").

Typically, categorical data is presented as percentages and proportions (e.g., 50 of 100 individuals in the sample, or 50%, were male). The statistic used to describe the center of their distribution is the *mode*, or the number of observations that appears most frequently. Variables that are described categorically are often called categorical variables.

Ordinal Data

If an inherent order exists among categories, the data is ordinal. For example:

How much education have you completed?	Circle one
Never finished high school	1
High school graduate, but no college	2
Some college	3
College graduate	4

Ordinal data is presented as percentages and proportions—for example, "20% of the sample are college graduates, but 30% never finished high school." The center of the distribution of responses is the *median*, or the observation that divides the distribution into halves. The median is equal to the 50th percentile. Variables that are described ordinally are often called ordinal variables.

Numerical Data

Numerical data can theoretically be described in infinitely small units. For example, age is a numerical variable; weight, length of survival, birth weight, and many laboratory values and standardized achievement test results are also numerical variables. Differences between numbers have meaning on a numerical scale (e.g., higher scores mean better achievement than lower scores, and a difference between 12 and 13 has the same meaning as a difference between 99 and 100). Numerical data is amenable to precision; that is, the evaluator can obtain data on age, for example, to the nearest second.

Numerical data may be *continuous*, such as height, weight, and age, or they may be *discrete*, such as numbers of visits to this clinic, number of absences from school. Means and standard deviations are used to summarize the values of numerical measures. Variables that are described numerically are often called either continuous or discrete variables.

Table 8.1 contrasts the three types of data.

SELECTING AN ANALYSIS METHOD

The analysis method is dependent on the following:

- The characteristics of the data collected for the independent variable. Is the data categorical, ordinal, or numerical?
- The number of independent variables.
- The characteristics of the data collected for the dependent variable. Is the data categorical, ordinal, or numerical?
- The number of dependent variables.
- Whether the design, sampling, and quality of the data meet the assumptions of the statistical method. These assumptions vary from method to method and are based on expectations about the nature and quality of the data and how they are distributed (normal or skewed).

Table 8.1 Categorical, Ordinal, and Numerical Data

Type of Data	Examples	Comments
Categorical	Ethnicity; gender	Observations belong to categories. Observations have no inherent order of importance. When data assumes two values (yes, I read history books; no, I don't read history books), it is termed *dichotomous*. Percentages and proportions are used to describe categorical data, and the mode is used to measure the midpoint.
Ordinal	Socioeconomic status (high, medium, low education; above, at, or below the poverty line); agreement with a statement (strongly agree, agree, disagree, strongly disagree)	Order exists among the categories; that is, observation 1 is higher in rank than observation 2. Percentages and proportions are used to describe ordinal data; the measure of the center of the distribution of the data is often the median.
Numerical	Continuous numerical scales (scores on a test of mental health status); age; height; length of survival Discrete numerical scales (number of visits to the school, number of falls)	Means and standard deviations are used to describe numerical data.

Example 8.1 shows the relationships among evaluation questions and hypotheses, independent and dependent variables, research design and sample, types of data, and data analysis. Note that in the justification, the evaluator discusses why the chosen statistical test is appropriate: The data meets the test's assumptions.

Example 8.1 Analyzing Evaluation Data: Connections among Questions, Designs, Samples, Measures, and Analysis

Evaluation question: Is quality of life satisfactory?

Hypothesis: Experimental and control program groups will not differ in quality of life. (The evaluators want to reject this hypothesis; the study design will enable them to determine if the hypothesis can be rejected rather than confirmed.)

Evidence: A statistically significant difference in quality-of-life favoring program versus control group participants.

Independent variable: Group membership (program participants versus controls).

Design: An experimental design with parallel controls.

Sampling: Eligible participants are assigned at random to experimental or control group; 150 participants are in each group (a statistically derived sample size).

Dependent variable: Quality of life.

Data: Group membership (categorical data: experimental or control), quality of life (continuous numerical data from the CARES Questionnaire, a 100-point survey in which higher scores mean better quality).

Analysis: A two-sample independent groups *t*-test.

t-test assumptions: Each group must have a sample size of 30, the two groups are independent.

Justification for the analysis: This *t*-test is appropriate in this case because the independent variable's data is categorical and the dependent variable's data is numerical. In Example 8.1, the assumptions of a *t*-test are met. These assumptions are that each group has a sample size of at least 30, the sizes of both groups are about equal, the two groups are independent (an assumption that is met most easily with a strong evaluation design and a high-quality data collection effort), and the data is normally distributed. (If one of these assumptions is seriously violated, other rigorous analytic methods should be used, such as the Wilcoxon rank-sum test, also called the Mann-Whitney U test. This test makes no assumption about the normality of the distribution; whereas the t is termed parametric, this test is one of a number called nonparametric.)

Unfortunately, no definitive rules can be set for all evaluations and their data. Table 8.2, however, provides a general guide to the selection of 15 of the most used statistical methods.

Table 8.2 General Guide to Statistical Data-Analytic Methods in Program Evaluation

Sample Questions	Type of Data: Independent Variable	Type of Data: Dependent Variable	Analytic Method
For questions with one independent and one dependent variable			
Do experimental and control patients differ in their use or failure to use mental health services?	Categorical: group (experimental and control)	Categorical: use of mental health services (used services or did not)	Chi-square; Fisher's exact test; relative risk (risk ratio); odds ratio
How do the experimental and control groups compare in their attitudes (measured by their scores on the Attitude Survey)?	Categorical (dichotomous): group (experimental and control)	Continuous (attitude survey scores)	Independent samples, t-test
How do teens in the U.S., Canada, and England compare in their attitudes to political engagement (measured by their scores on the Attitude Survey)?	Categorical (more than two values: U.S., Canada, and England)	Continuous (attitude survey scores)	One-way ANOVA (uses the F test)
Do high scores on the Attitude Survey predict high scores on the Knowledge Test?	Continuous (attitude survey scores)	Continuous (knowledge scores)	Regression (when neither variable is independent or dependent, use correlation)
For questions with two or more independent variables			
Do males and females in the experimental and control programs differ in whether they adhered to a diet?	Categorical (gender, group)	Categorical (adhered or did not adhere to a diet)	Log-linear regression
Do males and females with differing scores on the Knowledge Test differ in whether they adhered to a diet?	Categorical (gender) and continuous (knowledge scores)	Categorical and dichotomous (adhered or did not adhere to a diet)	Logistic regression
How do males and females in the experimental and control programs compare in their attitudes (measured by their scores on the Attitude Survey)?	Categorical (gender and group)	Continuous (attitude survey scores)	Analysis of variance (ANOVA)

(Continued)

Table 8.2 (Continued)

Sample Questions	Type of Data: Independent Variable	Type of Data: Dependent Variable	Analytic Method
How are age and income and years living in the community related to attitudes (measured by scores on the Attitude Survey)?	Continuous (age and income and years living in the community)	Continuous (attitude survey scores)	Multiple regression
How do males and females in the experimental and control programs compare in their attitudes (measured by their scores on the Attitude Survey) when their level of education is controlled for?	Categorical (gender and group) with possible confounding factors (such as education)	Continuous (attitude survey scores)	Analysis of covariance (ANCOVA)
For questions with two or more independent and dependent variables			
How do males and females in the experimental and control programs compare in their attitude and knowledge scores?	Categorical (gender and group)	Continuous (scores on two measures: attitudes and knowledge)	Multivariate analysis of variance (MANOVA)

Hypothesis Testing and *p* Values: Statistical Significance

Evaluators often compare two or more groups to find out if differences in outcome exist that favor a program; if differences are present, the evaluators examine the magnitude of those differences for significance. Consider Example 8.2.

Example 8.2 Comparing Two Groups

Evaluation question: Do participants improve in their knowledge of how to interpret food-label information in making dietary choices?

Hypothesis: No difference will be found in knowledge.

Evidence:

1. A statistically significant difference in knowledge between participants and nonparticipants must be found. The difference in scores must be at least 15 points.
2. If a 15-point difference is found, participants will be studied for two years to determine the extent to which the knowledge is retained. The scores must be maintained (no significant differences) over the two-year period.

Measurements: Knowledge is measured on the Dietary Choices Test, a 25-item self-administered test.

Analysis: A *t*-test will be used to compare the two groups in their knowledge. Scores will be computed a second time, and a *t*-test will be used to compare the average or mean differences over time.

In the evaluation described in Example 8.2, tests of statistical significance are called for twice: to compare participants and nonparticipants at one point in time and to compare the same participants' scores over time. In addition, the evaluators stipulate that for the scores to have practical meaning, a 15-point difference between participants and nonparticipants must be obtained and sustained.

With experience, program evaluators have found that statistical significance is sometimes insufficient evidence of a program's merit. With very large samples, for example, very small differences in numerical values (such as scores on an achievement test or laboratory values) can be statistically significant but have little practical, educational, or clinical meaning and may incur more costs than benefits.

In the evaluation presented in Example 8.2, the standard includes a 15-point difference in test scores. If the difference between scores is statistically significant but is only 10 points, then the program will not be considered significant in a practical sense.

Statistical significance and the p value

A statistically significant program evaluation effect is one that is probably due to a planned intervention rather than to some chance occurrence. To determine statistical significance, the evaluator restates the evaluation question ("Does a difference exist?") as a null hypothesis ("No difference exists") and presets the level of significance and the value that the test statistic must obtain to be significant. After this is completed, the calculations are performed. The following guidelines describe the steps the evaluator takes in conducting a hypothesis test and in determining statistical significance.

Guidelines for Hypothesis Testing, Statistical Significance, and *p* Values

1. *State the evaluation question as a null hypothesis.* The null hypothesis (H_0) is a statement that no difference exists between the averages or means of two groups. The following are typical null hypotheses in program evaluations:
   - No difference exists between the experimental program's average or mean score and the control program's mean score.
   - No difference exists between the sample's (the evaluation's participants) mean score and the population's (the population from which the participants were sampled) mean score.

   When evaluators find that a difference does not exist between means, they use the following terminology: "We failed to reject the null hypothesis." They do not say, "We accepted the null hypothesis." Failing to reject the null suggests that a difference probably exists between the means—say, between Program A's and Program B's average scores. Until the evaluators examine the data, however, they do not know if A is favored or B is. When the evaluators have no advance knowledge of which is better, they use a two-tailed hypothesis test. When they have an alternative hypothesis in mind—say, A is larger (better) than B—they use a one-tailed test. Before they can describe the properties of the test, other activities must take place.

2. *State the level of significance for the statistical test (e.g., the t-test) being used.* The level of significance, when chosen before the test is performed, is called the alpha value (denoted by the Greek letter alpha: α). The alpha gives the probability of rejecting the null hypothesis when it is true.
3. Tradition keeps the alpha value small—.05, .01, or .001—because among the last things an evaluator needs is to reject a null hypothesis when, in fact, it is true and there is no difference between group means.

   The *p* value is the probability that an observed result (or result of a statistical test) is due to chance (and not to the program). It is calculated *after* the statistical test. If the *p* value is less than alpha, then the null hypothesis is rejected.

Current practice requires the specification of exact *p* values. That is, if the obtained *p* is .03, the evaluator should report that *p* = .03 rather than *p* < .05. Reporting the approximate *p* was common practice before the widespread use of computers (when statistical tables were the primary source of probabilities). This practice has not been eradicated, however. The merit of using the exact values can be seen in that, without them, a finding of *p* = .06 may be viewed as not significant, whereas a finding of *p* = .05 will be.

4. *Determine the value that the test statistic must attain to be significant.* Such values can be found in statistical tables. For example, for the *z* distribution (a standard, normal distribution) with an alpha of .05 and a two-tailed test, tabular values (found in practically all statistics textbooks and online) show that the area of acceptance for the null hypothesis is the central 95% of the *z* distribution and that the areas of rejection are 2.5% of the area in each tail. The value of *z* (found in statistical tables and generated by statistical software) that defines these areas is −1.96 for the lower tail and +1.96 for the upper tail. If the test statistic is less than −1.96 or greater than +1.96, it will be rejected.

5. Perform the calculation. For more in the z distribution and z-scores, see https://study.com/academy/lesson/estimating-areas-under-the-normal-curve-using-z-scores-lesson-quiz.html.

Clinical or Practical Significance: Using Confidence Intervals

A confidence interval (CI) gives the range of values (such as statistical means) within which the "true" value of a statistical finding falls. For example, suppose students in a reading program take a test and, on average, get a score of 10. When a statistical analysis reveals a 95% confidence interval of 9.50–10.50 (or 9.50, 10.50), the evaluator can conclude that that there is a 95% probability that the true value falls somewhere within the range of 9.50 and 10.50.

Evaluation studies often use and report confidence intervals to express statistical significance. For example, suppose a program aims to improve young people's engagement in local politics. Suppose also that the evaluators of the program randomize participants into two groups: an experimental and a control. Further, consider that the statistical analysis shows an average 3% increase in engagement scores over a year (95% CI, 2%–6%), and the increase favors experimental program participants. The hypothetical evaluators can then reasonably conclude that the difference between groups is statistically significant because the CI does not contain 0% or no improvement. But you may ask: Is 3% a meaningful difference? Scores can be misleading. A 3% increase in scores from time 1 to time 2 may be quite different on a ten-item test from that on a 100-item test.

Evaluators can use confidence intervals to remedy this situation and provide more convincing evidence of program effectiveness, quality, and value than they might by relying on statistical significance alone.

Suppose the evaluators of the political engagement program determine that at least a 10% increase in scores is needed to prove the program's effectiveness. Suppose also that they find that the experimental program participants improve their scores by 11% (95% CI, 8%–12%). In this case, the evaluators can be 95% confident that the program to improve engagement was effective statistically and practically. Sometimes the results are ambiguous, however, and the results are not statistically significant although they appear to be clinically significant. This can occur if the confidence interval is wide, containing a large range of scores because of small sample size or imperfect measures.

Evaluation studies with strong designs and valid measures can often equate statistical and practical significance because they can count on the data's accuracy. Regardless of the method used to decide on significance, evidence of effectiveness, quality, and value should be set in advance. This is the ethical thing to do and the best way to ensure that the evaluation will be designed to uncover true and significant differences if they exist.

RISKS AND ODDS

Evaluators commonly assess risk and odds in evaluation studies. These are alternative ways of describing the likelihood that a particular outcome will occur. Suppose that you are conducting a survey to find out why a weight-loss program was not effective. You decide to survey the people in the program to find out the nature and characteristics of the problems they had with dieting. You find that out of every 100 people who have trouble dieting, 20 report frequent problems. To identify the risk of a person having frequent problems, you divide the number of individuals reporting frequent problems by the number you are studying, or 20/100: The risk is 0.20.

The odds of a person having frequent problems are calculated differently. To get the odds, you subtract the number of persons with frequent problems (20) from the total (100) and use the result (80) as the denominator. Thus, the odds of having frequent problems with dieting are 20/80, or 0.25. Table 8.3 shows the difference between risk and odds.

Because assessing risk and calculating odds are really just different ways of talking about the same relationship, risk can be derived from odds, and vice versa. We can convert risk to odds by dividing it by 1 minus the risk, and we can convert odds to risk by dividing odds by 1 plus the odds:

$$\text{Odds} = \text{Risk}/(1 - \text{Risk}).$$

$$\text{Risk} = \text{Odds}/(1 + \text{Odds}).$$

When an outcome is infrequent, little difference exists in numerical values between odds and risk. When the outcome is frequent, however, differences emerge. If, for instance, 20 of 100 people have frequent problems following a diet, the risk and odds are similar: 0.20 and 0.25, respectively. If 90 of 100 people have frequent problems, then the risk is 0.90 and the odds are 9.00.

Odds Ratios and Relative Risk

Evaluators often use *odds ratios* to compare categorical dependent variables between groups. Odds ratios allow an evaluator to estimate the strength of the relationship between

Table 8.3 Risk and Odds, Compared and Contrasted

Number of Persons with Outcome	Risk	Odds
20 of 100	20/100 = 0.20	20/80 = 0.25
40 of 100	40/100 = 0.40	40/60 = 0.66
50 of 100	50/100 = 0.50	50/50 = 1.00
90 of 100	90/100 = 0.90	90/10 = 9.00

variables. For example, suppose that you have evidence that people who have trouble dieting also do not eat breakfast. (You have reason to believe that people who don't eat breakfast often decide to snack before lunchtime.) You want to check out the strength of the relationship between not eating breakfast and subsequent problems with keeping to a diet. You put together two groups of people: those who have problems adhering to a diet and those who do not. You ask them all, "Do you eat breakfast?" Their response choices are categorical: yes or no.

To analyze the responses, you might create a 2 × 2 table such as the following:

	Trouble Adhering to Diet?	
	Yes	No
No Breakfast? Yes	A	B
No	C	D

This is a 2 × 2 table because it has two variables with two levels: breakfast (yes or no) and problems adhering (yes or no). Notice that the table has four cells for data entry. The two variables, "no breakfast" and "problems adhering," are categorical variables.

If you were interested only in whether statistical differences exist in the numbers of people in each of the cells, you could use the chi-square test. A chi-square test will not tell you about the strength of the relationship between the variables, however; it will only allow you to infer differences. An odds ratio, in contrast, will allow you to say something like this: "The odds of having problems adhering to a diet are greater (or lesser) among people who eat (or do not eat) breakfast."

The odds ratio is used in evaluations that use case control designs. In such evaluations, the researcher decides how many "cases" (e.g., people who have problems) and "controls" (e.g., people who do not have problems) to include in the sample. To calculate the odds ratio, the evaluator counts how many in each group have the "risk factor" (e.g., no breakfast) and divides the odds of having the risk factor among the cases by the odds of having the risk factor among the controls.

Odds ratios are integral components of other statistical methods. Analytic software programs that do logistic regressions or interpret them automatically yield odds ratios. Example 8.3 gives the formula for the odds ratio.

Example 8.3 The Formula for the Odds Ratio

Risk Factor Present?

Risk Factor Present?	Case	Control	Total
Yes	A	B	a + b
No	C	D	c + d
Total	a + c	b + d	n

Example 8.4 illustrates how this formula works.

Example 8.4 The Odds Ratio in Action

Suppose that you are interested in the relationship between not eating breakfast (the risk factor) and trouble adhering to a diet. You ask this question: When compared with people who eat breakfast, what is the likelihood that people who do not will have trouble adhering to a weight-loss diet?

You identify 400 people who have trouble adhering to a diet and 400 who do not. You find that among all people with problems, 100 do not eat breakfast and 300 do. Among people without problems, 50 do not eat breakfast. To compare the odds of problems between the two groups, you put the data into a 2 × 2 table:

Problems Keeping to a Diet

No Breakfast	Case	Control	Total
Yes	100	50	150
No	300	400	700
Total	400	450	850

The odds ratio (OR) is calculated as follows:

$$OR = ad/bc = 100 \times 400/50 \times 300 = 40,000/15,000 = 2.67.$$

The odds of being exposed to the risk factor (no breakfast) are 2.67 higher for people in the sample who have problems adhering to a weight-loss diet than for people who do not have such problems. The answer to your question is that people who do not eat breakfast are 2.67 times more likely to encounter problems adhering to a diet than people who eat breakfast.

Evaluators also use *risk ratios* to examine the strength of the relationship between two categorical variables, but this method for studying the relationship is different from calculating odds ratios. Risk ratios are calculated for evaluations using a cohort design (for more on cohort designs, see Chapter 3). Suppose that you want to determine how likely it is that people who do not eat breakfast have trouble adhering to a weight-loss diet. First you pick the cohort—in this situation, people with problems adhering to a diet. Then you select a period of time to observe them—say, 12 months. At the end of the 12 months, you count the number of people who had adherence problems and the number of people who did not. Do these numbers differ? If so, was a greater risk likely for people who did not eat breakfast?

When you rely on cohort designs to calculate risk ratios (also called *relative risk* or *likelihood ratios*), you have no control over how many people are in each group. Obviously, you cannot control the number of people in the study group who develop problems, although you do have control over the number of people in your study group. The evaluator who uses a case control design has control over the numbers of people who have and who do not have the problem. He or she can say: "I will have 100 cases and 100 controls." It may take the case control evaluator more or less than 12 months to identify enough cases for each group. In technical terms, the risk ratio is the ratio of the incidence of "disease" (e.g., problems adhering to a diet) among the "exposed" (people who do not eat breakfast) to the incidence of "disease" among the "nonexposed" (people who do eat breakfast). Incidence rates can be estimated only prospectively.

In a case control study, you cannot estimate the probability of having a problem because you, the evaluator, have determined in advance how many people are in the cases and how many are in the controls. All you can do is determine the probability of having the risk factor. This is unusual given that normally evaluators are concerned with finding out the probability of having the problem, not the risk for the problem. However, when you compare odds in an odds ratio, you will find that the ratio of the odds for having the risk factor is identical to the ratio of odds for having the disease or problem. Thus, you can calculate the same odds ratio for a case control as for a cohort study or randomized controlled trial. It doesn't matter which variable is independent and which is dependent—the odds ratio will have exactly the same value. This is not true of risk ratios, and so researchers find odds ratios an excellent way to answer questions or test hypotheses involving categorical dependent variables between groups defined by categorical independent variables.

QUALITATIVE EVALUATION DATA: CONTENT ANALYSIS

Content analysis is a method for analyzing qualitative information. Qualitative information differs from statistical data in that the endpoints are narratives and personal observations rather than numbers or test results like p values. The evaluator may collect qualitative information directly from people by asking them questions about their knowledge, attitudes, and behavior, or indirectly, through observations of their behavior. The behavior may be online (measuring how often a web page is visited or how frequently an article is downloaded), via social media (how many "likes" a video has), and in person (how many informal groups of children are created in a school yard during lunch period). Survey questionnaires often ask people to comment about events using their own words as opposed to having them react to preset questions and response choices.

Analyzing qualitative data requires the evaluator to pore over the respondents' written or verbal comments to look for ideas or *themes* that appear repeatedly across groups (experimental and control) and subgroups (teens 14 and under versus teens 15 and older). Once the themes are identified, they are coded, which allows them to be entered into a database, counted, and compared.

Another familiar type of qualitative data comes from observations of people. For example, two members of an evaluation team might spend a month observing patients as they arrive at a hospital's emergency department to determine what happens to them as they wait to be seen by health professionals. The observers would then compare notes and summarize their findings.

Evaluators might also obtain qualitative data from documents and from various forms of media that were produced for other purposes. For instance, suppose that you are part of a program planning and evaluation team that wants to start an antismoking media campaign in a particular community. A first step is to examine how stories about smoking and health have been handled across all media.

Of the several types of media, you decide to restrict your review of stories about smoking and health to three social media sites. As in any analysis, you also must be concerned with research design, sampling, and analysis. What time period should your review cover? The past year? Three years? How should you define and code each entry? Which data-analytic methods are appropriate for comparing the number and types of entries over time?

You might hypothesize that the number of references to the harmful effects of smoking increased significantly in the three sites from 2019 to 2023, but that the number of references has remained relatively constant since that time. You can use content analysis methods to test these hypotheses and to answer your research questions.

There are five main activities involved in conducting a content analysis:

1. Assembling the data
2. Learning the contents of the data
3. Creating a codebook or data dictionary
4. Entering and cleaning the data
5. Doing the analysis

Assembling the Data

Qualitative data often takes the form of a great many pages of notes and interview transcripts. Unsorted data is the foundation of a qualitative database. It is not the same as the database, and, on its own, it is not interpretable or amenable to analysis.

In addition to transcripts of individual and group interviews and field notes from observations, qualitative data includes participants' responses to open-ended survey questions and reviews of written, spoken, and filmed materials.

Transcripts are written, printed, or recorded accounts of every word spoken in interviews or by observed individuals during data collection. Producing a transcript can take a great deal of time. For example, a verbatim report of a typical discussion among eight people during a 90-minute group interview may result in 50 or more pages of transcript text.

Of course, not all data in a complete transcript is necessarily relevant. Sometimes people get sidetracked during a discussion: They tell jokes, change the subject, and so on, and reviewing these digressions may be unnecessary. Because producing complete transcripts is so time-consuming, and because they often contain irrelevant information, some evaluators rely on abridged transcripts. It should be noted, however, that by using abridged transcripts, an evaluator may run the risk of excluding important information. Diversionary acts may be a signal of boredom with the discussion or of poor leadership, and both factors may be important for the evaluators to consider.

Written transcripts do not capture the expressions on people's faces during a discussion, nor do they adequately describe the passion with which some people state their positions. Because of this, transcripts are often supplemented by audio and visual documentation.

Evaluators sometimes use portions of the visual and audio records from their studies in their evaluation reports to illustrate the findings and lend a "human" touch to the reports' words and statistics. Evaluators should be aware, however, that any use of participants' words, voices, emails, texts, or visual images to justify or explain the research findings or recommendations may raise legal and ethical questions. Participants must be given the opportunity to consent to the use of their words and visual images in advance of data collection. They should be told where and under what circumstances the information will be used and what the risks and benefits of use are.

Field notes are the notes taken by observers or interviewers "in the field"—that is, while they are conducting observations or interviews. Transcribing and sorting through field notes is an onerous process. The evaluator must review the notes and fill in any missing information, which requires remembering what was said or done, when, and by whom. Some people have great memories; others are less fortunate. Some observers and interviewers take better notes than others. It is preferable to have two or more observers taking notes in any given setting, so that the evaluator can compare their findings to estimate interrater reliability (for more on interrater reliability, see Chapter 6).

Having two note takers or observers may also reduce the amount of recall needed to assemble a complete set of data because if one observer forgets who did what to whom, the other may have recorded the information in detail. Using two or more observers in a setting can, however, increase a study's personnel costs. Also, with two or more observers, disagreement is inevitable. The need for a third person to arbitrate when disagreements occur also increases personnel costs, as well as the time needed to organize notes and observations.

Focus groups are targeted discussion groups. To be effective, a focus group must be led by a skilled moderator, an individual who is able to focus the group's attention on a specific topic. Note takers are often employed to record focus group discussions because the moderators are too busy keeping group members on track to take notes as well. However, even skilled note takers may leave out a great deal of information due to the difficulty of capturing every speaker's point. Because of the fear of losing vital information, evaluators usually record focus group discussions, again raising legal and privacy concerns. Voice recognition software is available that can eliminate some of the difficulties of transcribing and interpreting notes.

Learning the Contents of the Data

The evaluator's second step in content analysis is to become extremely familiar with the data that has been collected. Evaluators must understand the data thoroughly before they can assign it codes in anticipation of data entry and analysis. Learning the contents of the data can mean reading through hundreds of recorded pages of text, watching videotapes, and listening to audiotapes for days or even weeks. Becoming reacquainted with the discussion in a single group interview, for example, may require a full day of the evaluator's time, and transcribing one hour's worth of audiotape may take four to eight hours.

Creating a Codebook or Data Dictionary

Surveys with closed (or closed-ended) questions assign codes or values in advance of data collection. Surveys with open-ended questions assign codes after the data is collected. This is illustrated in Example 8.5.

Example 8.5 Coding Closed and Open-Ended Questions

Closed Questions

The following are excerpts from a survey of visits to a clinic made by new mothers as part of an evaluation of the effectiveness of a program to prevent postpartum depression.

Question 5. Did the mother visit the clinic within 2 weeks of delivery? (postpartum)

Yes   ❑ (1)
No   ❑ (0)
No data   ❑ (.a)

Question 7. Did the mother visit the clinic within 6 weeks of delivery? (well visit)

Yes   ❑ (1)
No   ❑ (0)
No data   ❑ (.a)

A corresponding portion of a codebook for this survey appears as follows:

Variable Number	Variable Number	Description and Comments
1.	PROJID	A five-digit ID project code
2.	INDIVID	A four-digit ID individual code
3.	DLIVDATE	Enter month/day/year using two digits for each segment. Example: May 20, 2023=05202023
4.	FOLLDATE	Use same procedure as for DLIVDATE
5.	POSPARVIS	No = 0; Yes = 1; use. a if missing
6.	VISTDATE	Follow DLIVDATE procedure. If POSPARVIS = No, use 0; use. a if missing
7.	WELVISIT	No = 0; Yes= 1; use. a if missing

Open-Ended Questions

The following are excerpts from a summarized transcript of a group interview discussion among participants in an evaluation of a program to prevent postpartum depression in new mothers.

Theme	Code
Identified common depressive symptoms but did not always conceptualize them as an illness (depression)	1
Acknowledged role of environmental stress (environment)	2
Pointed to need for new knowledge about counseling (knowledge)	3
Wanted to help themselves but felt impaired by depression and lack of information (depression; knowledge)	1 and 3
Felt that having someone to talk to in a confidential manner, to be able to "unburden oneself," would be helpful (counseling)	4
Believed counselor might be able to help them solve their own problems, change their negative thoughts and behaviors, have a more positive outlook (counseling)	4

Entering and Cleaning the Data

In content analysis, data entry involves organizing and storing the contents of transcripts and notes. Data may be entered and organized by person, place, observation, quotation, or some other feature. If you are conducting a very small program evaluation, you might be tempted to organize such data on index cards. However, better options for storage include spreadsheets, database management programs, and word-processing programs. Software designed specifically for qualitative analysis is also available, but it may be costly, and it requires some training to be used properly.

Cleaning the data may mean deciding on which data to discard. Why would anyone discard data? Sometimes evaluators must discard data because it is indecipherable (e.g., incomplete recordings or unreadable notes) or irrelevant. When evaluators elect to discard data, they must create rules regarding what to do about lost or missing data.

How will the lost data be handled? How much will the absence of data influence the conclusions that can be drawn? When data is missing, the evaluator must be sure to discuss the implications of this fact in the evaluation report.

Once the data is cleaned and its strengths and weaknesses are understood, it can be organized into a database. Only a clean database stands a chance of producing reliable information. Inconsistent and incomprehensible information is invalid and biased.

Obtaining a clean database is an objective shared by all evaluators, whether their data collection methods are qualitative or statistical. Accomplishing this objective is extremely time-consuming, and evaluators using qualitative data collection should plan adequate time for this major task regardless of the size of the evaluation.

Doing the Analysis

The final step is doing the analysis. One approach to the analysis involves asking respondents to give their views without prompting, whereas another approach involves prompting in the form of mentioning specific topics or themes. Example 8.6 shows how a content analysis with prompting might work.

Example 8.6 Content Analysis and Barriers to Attendance at Depression Therapy Classes

Evaluation data collection: Structured interview with 200 new mothers.

Purpose: To discover barriers to attendance at depression therapy classes.

Premise: Barriers include lack of transportation, lack of childcare for older children, inability to get off from work, lack of motivation (don't think they need the classes).

Question: Which of the following [the barriers are listed] is the most important reason why you or other mothers might not be able to attend parenting classes?

Analysis: Count each time a particular barrier (e.g., lack of transportation) is chosen as the most important reason.

Results:

Barriers	50 Mothers 25 Years of Age and Younger	150 Mothers 26 Years of Age and Older
Lack of transportation	15*	86
Lack of childcare	20	81
Inability to get off from work	5	17
Doesn't need classes	40	16

* The number in each cell represents the number of times that barrier is mentioned.

Conclusions: Overall, lack of childcare and lack of transportation are the most frequently mentioned reasons for not attending classes. Older and younger women differed in their barriers, with younger women believing strongly that they don't need classes. A greater number of older women than younger women cited lack of transportation as a barrier. Inability to get off from work was not cited frequently by either age group.

Prompting to collect evaluation information means identifying preselected themes. The evaluator must derive such themes from the research literature and from experience. If you were to prompt the mothers in Example 8.6 with preselected themes, you might ask them to come together in a group interview or focus group to answer questions like these: How important is lack of transportation (childcare, inability to get off work) as a reason for your coming or not coming to classes? What other reasons can you think of that might help us understand why women might choose to stay away from classes? After the group session, you would analyze the data by reviewing the transcript of the interview and counting the number of times the participants cited each of the barriers.

META-ANALYSIS

Meta-analysis is a statistical method for combining the findings of multiple studies all of which address the same research question. Each study's research question and the evaluation's research question must be identical for the meta-analysis to be valid. The idea behind meta-analysis is that the larger numbers obtained from combining or "pooling" the results of many studies have greater statistical power and generalizability than the results of any individual study on its own.

Meta-analysis provides a quantitative alternative to a traditional literature review in which experts use judgment and intuition to reach conclusions about the merits of a program or, alternatively, base their conclusions on a count of the number of positive versus negative and inconclusive studies.

Each study in a meta-analysis almost always contains some bias or error because of imperfect designs and measures, and many differ from one another in their samples and settings. The meta-analysis must use statistical methods to account for the bias and heterogeneity, or pooling the results is not possible. This accounting is a major challenge to meta-analysis statisticians and to the subsequent validity of the findings. The accuracy of a meta-analysis depends entirely on the quality of the literature included in it and the statistical methods used to control bias.

Meta-analysis methods are continually advancing. Techniques for cumulative meta-analyses, for example, permit the identification of the year when the combined results of multiple studies first achieved a given level of statistical significance. The technique also reveals whether the temporal trend seems to be leaning toward superiority of one program or intervention or another, and it allows assessment of the impact of each new study on the pooled estimate of the treatment effect.

SUMMARY AND TRANSITION TO THE NEXT CHAPTER ON EVALUATION REPORTS

This chapter discussed data analysis methods that are particularly useful in program evaluations. Before choosing a method, the evaluator must determine the number of variables that will be studied as well as the characteristics and distribution of the data. When using tests of significance as evidence of program effectiveness, quality, and value, the evaluator must decide on clinical or practical as well as statistical meaning, and the decision should be made in advance of the analysis.

The next chapter discusses written and oral evaluation reports. It describes the contents of written reports, including objectives, methods, results, conclusions, discussion, and recommendations. Special emphasis is placed on the use of tables and figures to present data. The chapter also explains the contents of a report's abstract or concise overview (typically about 250 words). Published evaluation reports are required to conform to standard reporting guidelines such as CONSORT and TREND. Each of these is discussed in the next chapter.

Because evaluation reporting is often oral, the chapter also provides guidelines for the preparation of oral presentations and posters.

EXERCISES: CHAPTER 8

Exercise 1

Directions

For each of the following situations, describe the independent and dependent variables and determine whether they will be described with categorical, ordinal, or numerical data.

Situation	Describe the independent and dependent variables	Is the data categorical, ordinal, or numerical?
Patients in the experimental and control groups tell whether painkillers give complete, moderate, or very little relief.		
Participants in the program are grouped according to whether they are severely, moderately, or marginally depressed and are given a survey of anxiety that is scored from 1 to 9.		
Children are chosen for evaluation according to whether they have had all recommended vaccinations; they are followed for five years, and their health status is monitored.		
Men and women with stage 1, 2, and 3 of a disease are compared in quality of life as measured by scores ranging from 1 to 50 that are obtained from standardized observations.		

Exercise 2

Directions

Use the following information to select and justify a data analysis method.

Evaluation question: After program participation, is domestic violence decreased?
Evidence: A statistically significant difference in domestic violence is found between families who have participated in the experimental program and families in the control program.
Independent variable: Group or program membership (experimental versus control).
Design: An experimental design with parallel controls.
Sampling: Eligible participants are assigned at random to either an experimental group or a control group; 100 participants are in each group (a statistically derived sample size).
Dependent variable: Domestic violence.
Data: Data on domestic violence will come from the DONT Survey, a 50-point measure in which lower scores mean less violence.

Exercise 3

Directions

Suppose that the evaluation of the program to reduce domestic violence described in Exercise 2 is concerned about comparing younger and older persons in the experimental and control groups. Assuming the use of the DONT Survey, which produces continuous scores, which statistical method would be appropriate? Explain.

SUGGESTED READING

Braitman, L.E. (1991). Confidence intervals assess both clinical and statistical significance. *Annals of Internal Medicine, 114,* 515–517.

Examples of Meta-Analyses

Aghasi, M., Golzarand, M., Shab-Bidar, S., Aminianfar, A., Omidian, M., & Taheri, F. (2019). Dairy intake and acne development: A meta-analysis of observational studies. *Clinical Nutrition (Edinburgh, Scotland), 38*(3): 1067–1075.

Caldwell, D.M., Davies, S.R, Hetrick SE, et al. (2019). School-based interventions to prevent anxiety and depression in children and young people: A systematic review and network meta-analysis. *The Lancet Psychiatry, 6*(12): 1011–1020.

Cortese, S., Adamo, N., Del Giovane, C., et al. (2018). Comparative efficacy and tolerability of medications for attention-deficit hyperactivity disorder in children, adolescents, and adults: A systematic review and network meta-analysis. *The Lancet Psychiatry, 5*(9): 727–738.

Li, F., Lu, H., Zhang, Q., et al. (2021). Impact of COVID-19 on female fertility: A systematic review and meta-analysis protocol. *BMJ Open, 11*(2): e045524.

Siafis, S., Çıray, O., Wu, H., et al. (2022). Pharmacological and dietary-supplement treatments for autism spectrum disorder: A systematic review and network meta-analysis. *Molecular Autism, 13*(1): 10.

Suggested Websites

Zedstatistics—Teach me STATISTICS in half an hour! Seriously
www.youtube.com/watch?v=kyjlxsLW1Is

Cochrane Training
https://training.cochrane.org

ANSWERS TO EXERCISES: CHAPTER 8

Exercise 1

Situation	Describe the independent and dependent variables	Is the data nominal, ordinal, or numerical?
Patients in the experimental and control group tell if painkillers give complete, moderate, or very little relief.	Independent variable: group Dependent variable: pain relief	Independent variable: nominal Dependent variable: ordinal
Participants in the program are grouped according to whether they are severely, moderately, or marginally depressed and are given a survey of anxiety that is scored from 1 to 9.	Independent variable: depressed patients in the program Dependent variable: anxiety	Independent variable: ordinal Dependent variable: numerical
Children are chosen for the evaluation according to whether they have had all recommended vaccinations; they are followed for five years, and their health status is monitored.	Independent variable: having or not having recommended the vaccinations Dependent variable: health status	Independent variable: nominal Dependent variable: not enough information to tell
Men and women with stage 1, 2, and 3 of a disease are compared in quality of life as measured by scores ranging from 1 to 50 that are obtained from standardized observations.	Independent variable: gender and stage of disease Dependent variable: quality of life	Independent variables: nominal and ordinal Dependent variable: numerical

Exercise 2

Analysis: A two-sample independent groups *t*-test

Justification for the analysis: This t-test is appropriate when the independent variable is measured on a nominal scale and the dependent variable is measured on a numerical scale. In this case, the assumptions of a *t*-test are met. These assumptions are that each group has a sample size of at least 30, the two groups are about equal in size, and the two groups are independent.

Exercise 3

If the evaluation aims to find out how younger and older persons in the experimental and control groups compare in amount of domestic violence, and presuming that the statistical assumptions are met, then analysis of variance is an appropriate technique.

CHAPTER 9 | EVALUATION REPORTS

PURPOSE OF CHAPTER 9

This chapter explains how to prepare a transparent evaluation report. A transparent report provides a detailed and accurate explanation of the evaluation's purposes, methods, and conclusions. Transparency improves with the use of standardized reporting checklists such as the Consolidated Standards of Reporting Trials (CONSORT Statement) and Transparent Reporting of Evaluations with Nonrandomized Designs (TREND).

Evaluation reports take the form of printed or online manuscripts, oral presentations, or posters. The chapter first discusses how to prepare manuscripts and describes the figures and tables you need to show results. Next, the chapter examines oral reports and offers recommendations for preparing slides and posters that are useful for online or in-person presentations.

A READER'S GUIDE TO CHAPTER 9

DOI: 10.4324/9781032635071-9

THE WRITTEN EVALUATION REPORT

An evaluation report describes and synthesizes all evaluation purposes, methods, results, conclusions, and recommendations The report also include a statement of caution about the validity of the conclusions because of any potential biases due to such factors as faulty research designs or failures to monitor program implementation. Written evaluation reports may be published as monographs, papers, and journal articles. The information presented in them may be reported upon in person or online via video conference sharing or video. Oral (and sometimes written) reports often rely on slide presentations. All evaluation reports use figures, tables, and photos; some may also incorporate audio and visual data. A useful evaluation report provides enough information so that at least two interested individuals who read or listen to the report independently agree on the evaluation's purposes, methods, and conclusions.

If an evaluation report (regardless of the form it takes) is to be submitted to a funding organization, such as a foundation, trust, or government agency, the composition and format of the report are likely to be set by that organization. In many cases, however, evaluators are on their own in deciding on the length and content of their reports. Most written and readable program evaluation reports are somewhere between 2,500 and 15,000 words in length—that is, 15 to 60 double-spaced printed pages (using common fonts such as Arial and Times New Roman, 11- to 12-point type, and one-inch margins).

In addition to the text, evaluation reports include lists of relevant bibliographic references as well as tables and figures (e.g., photographs, graphs) to illustrate evaluation findings; usually, no more than ten tables and ten figures are needed. In addition, an abstract of approximately 250 words and a summary of up to 15 pages are often helpful. Very long reports are rarely read. Evaluators who produce long reports should always make sure that their executive summaries are well done, because most people will focus on those.

Evaluation reports sometimes post online working documents such as résumés, project worksheets, survey response frequencies, complex mathematical calculations, copies of measures (such as survey questionnaires or literature review forms), organizational charts, memorandums, training materials, videos, and project planning documents.

Example 9.1 gives the table of contents for an evaluation report on an 18-month program combining diet and exercise to improve health status and quality of life for persons 75 years of age or older.

Example 9.1 Sample Table of Contents for a Report: An Evaluation of the Living-at-Home Program for Elders (18-Month Program to Improve Health Status and Quality of Life for People 75+ Years)

Abstract: 250 words
Summary: 8 pages
Text of report: 41 pages

    D. Outcome Measures
       1. Reliability and validity of measures of quality of life, health, and cost-effectiveness
       2. Quality assurance system for the data collection
    E. Analysis

(In this section, the evaluators cite and justify the specific method used to test each hypothesis or answer each evaluation question. For example: "To compare men and women in their health, we used a t-test, and to predict who benefited most from participation in the experimental program, we relied on stepwise multiple regressions.")

  III. Results (15 pages)
    A. Response rates (such as how many eligible men and women agreed to participate in the evaluation; how many completed the entire program; how many individuals completed all data collection requirements). This information can be presented in a flow chart
    B. Demographic and other descriptive characteristics (for the experimental and control groups: numbers and percentages of men and women; numbers and percentages under 65 to 75 years of age, 76 to 85, and 85 and older; numbers and percentages choosing each of the two health care staffing models)
    C. Effectiveness: Quality of Life and Health Status
    D. Cost-Effectiveness of Two Staffing Models of Care
  IV. Conclusions (7 pages)
   V. Limitations on Interpretation
  VI. Recommendations (2 pages)
 VII. Tables and Figures
    A. Table 1. Demographic Characteristics of Participants
    B. Table 2. Health Outcomes and Quality of Life for Men and Women with Varying Levels of Illness
    C. Table 3. Costs of Three Clinic Staffing Models
    D. Figure 1. Flowchart: How Participants Were Assigned to Groups by "Cluster"
VIII. Online Supplements/Appendixes
    A. Copies of all measures
    B. Calculations linking costs and effectiveness
    C. Final calculations of sample size
    D. Testimony from program participants regarding their satisfaction with participation in the experimental program
    E. Informed consent statements
    F. List of panel participants and affiliations
    G. Training materials for all data collection
    H. Data collection quality assurance plan

Suppose that the Living-at-Home Program whose report is outlined in Example 9.1 works this way:

- *Program:* The members of an experimental group of older adults who still live at home receive the diet and exercise program, whereas older adults in another living-at-home group do not. Participants in the evaluation who need medical services choose freely between two clinics offering differing models of care, one staffed primarily by physicians and the other staffed primarily by nurses.
- *Assignment to study groups:* Participants are randomly assigned to the experimental or control programs according to the streets on which they live. That is, participants living on Street A are randomly assigned, as are participants living on Streets B, C, and so on.
- *Main outcomes:* (a) Whether program participation makes a difference in the health and quality of life of older men and women and the role of patient mix in making those differences and (b) the cost-effectiveness of the two models of health care delivery.

COMPOSITION OF THE REPORT

Introduction

The introduction to a program evaluation report has three components: (a) a description of the problem, (b) an explanation of how the experimental program is to solve it, and (c) a list of questions that the evaluation plans to answer about program effectiveness, quality, and value. Example 9.2 illustrates the contents of the introduction to a written report.

Example 9.2 Contents of the Introduction to a Written Evaluation Report

Your written evaluation report's introduction should include information on the following:

1. *The problem:* Describe the problem that the program and its evaluation are designed to solve. In the description, tell how many people are affected by the problem and what its human and financial costs are. Cite the literature or other valid sources to defend your estimates of the importance and costs of the problem.
2. *The program:* Give an overview of the program's objectives and activities and any unique features (such as its size, location, and number and types of participants). If the program is modelled on some other intervention, describe the similarities and differences, and cite supporting references.
3. *The evaluation:* State the objectives of the evaluation, justify the choice of evaluation questions and the evidence of program effectiveness, quality, and value. If you used an evaluation framework to guide planning and evaluation, describe it and its use in the evaluation. Establish the connections among the general problem, the objectives of the program, and the evaluation. That is, tell how the evaluation provides knowledge about the program and provides new knowledge about the problem, as in the following example of the evaluation of a home health care program for older adults. (Box)

Sample Introduction

The purpose of this evaluation is to identify whether community-dwelling elderly who participated in a home health care program improved in their health and quality of life. Participants were randomly assigned to an experimental or a control group. Because evidence exists that home health care can improve social, emotional, and physical functioning in the elderly [references regarding the potential benefits of home health care should have been cited in the first part of the introduction], we asked about the effectiveness of the program for men and women of differing ages and levels of medical and social problems and the nature, characteristics, and costs of effective home health services. Using the literature as a basis for deciding upon evidence of effectiveness, we hypothesized that the experimental group would see greater improvements than the control, and that it would not be any costlier.

Methods

The methods section of the report should define terms and describe the program or interventions, design, setting, participants, sample, measures, analysis, results, conclusions, and limitations on interpretation. Tables and figures help the reader understand the evaluation and its findings.

- *The program:* Describe the experimental and comparison programs, carefully distinguishing between them. How long did each participate in the evaluation? If you prepared protocols to standardize the implementation of the programs, describe them and any training in the use of the protocols that took place.
- *Definitions:* Define all potentially misleading terms, such as quality of life, behavior, attitudes, knowledge, high risk, value, and efficiency.

- *Design:* Tell whether the evaluation used an experimental or observational design. If the design was experimental, specify the type (e.g., parallel controls, in which participants are randomly assigned to experimental and control groups).
- *Setting:* Report on where the evaluation data was collected. You might include the geography (e.g., name of city and state or country), the locale (e.g., urban versus rural), and the site (e.g., clinic, community).
- *Participants:* Give the inclusion and exclusion criteria for participation in the evaluation. Tell whether the participants were randomly selected and randomly assigned.
- *Sampling.* Explain how the sample sizes were determined. Provide a flow chart that describes how the final sample came about. Start with the number of people who were eligible and the number who were approached and agreed to participate. Discuss the number who completed all data collection.
- *Measures:* Describe each outcome and the characteristics of the data collection measures for the main evaluation questions. Who administered the measure? Was training required? Is the measure reliable? Is it valid? How much time is required to complete the measure? How many questions does it contain? How were they selected? If appropriate, cite the theory behind the choice of questions or the other measures on which they were based. How is the measure scored?
- *Analysis:* Check each evaluation question for the main variables. Then, for the main variables, describe and justify the analytic method. Have you used any unusual methods in the analysis? If so, you should describe them. Name the statistical package used in case other evaluators want to perform a similar analysis using the same setup. If you have used a relatively new or complex data-analytic method, provide references to justify using it.
- *Results:* The results section of the report presents the results of the process or implementation evaluation and the statistical analyses. All response rates should appear in this section, along with descriptions of the evaluation participants' characteristics.
- This section should include a comparison of the individuals who agreed to participate with those who refused or did not complete the entire program or provide complete data. The results for each major evaluation question and its sub-questions also appear in this section. For example, if one of your main questions asks whether patients' quality of life improves, you should present the results for that question. You might also provide data on the types of individuals (e.g., older men, sicker patients) for whom the program was most and least effective in terms of quality of life.

Tables and figures are almost always used in evaluation reports to summarize the study's results.

- *Conclusions or Discussion*: The conclusions or discussion section of the evaluation report should tell readers what the results mean. Is the program effective? With whom does it work best? How would you rate its quality? Is the program cost-effective? Does it have value?
- *Limitations*: What are the potential biases? Was the dropout rate larger than anticipated? Were the results based on analysis of self-administered surveys and not behavior? Did the results meet the criterion of statistical significance but fail to meet that of clinical or practical significance?

Tables and Figures

Tables and figures are frequently used to help readers understand the evaluation's methods and results. The most often used are flow charts describing the recruitment and retention of an evaluation's participants, tables depicting the participant's demographic and other relevant characteristics, and tables describing the evaluation's statistical results.

Figure 9.1 illustrates the use of a flow chart to describe the selection and retention of patients in an online education program called "Wise Drinking as We Age." As can be seen from the flow chart, 172 of 381 eligible people gave their informed consent to join

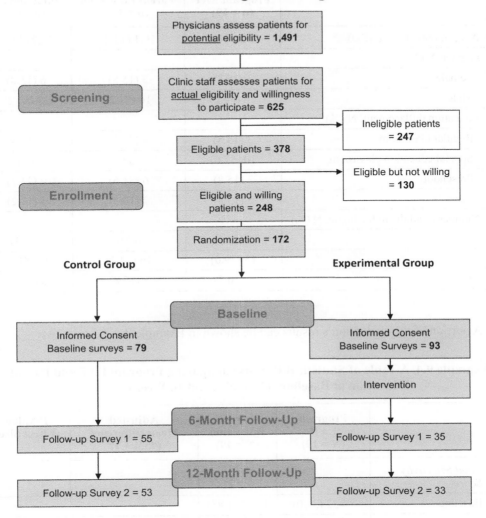

Figure 9.1 Flow Diagram of Enrollment into the Evaluation of Wise Drinking as We Age

the evaluation, but a total of 86 completed all study activities. The dropout rate was higher in the experimental than in the control group. High numbers of people lost to follow up are common in studies of difficult subjects like drinking and aging. Nevertheless, the low retention rate clearly confers limitations on the study's findings, and the retained sample of participants may be very different from the general population in factors such as motivation or education.

Example 9.3 shows a typical "Table 1" in an evaluation report which describes pertinent demographic and other characteristics of the evaluation sample at baseline. In this case, the sample consists of special needs children and their parents. The evaluation compares two programs to improve the eating habits of special needs children. The programs are different, with Program EAT focused on children and Program Education designed for parents.

Example 9.3 Baseline Characteristics by Program Group

	Program EAT (n = 19)	Parent Education (n = 19)	Total Sample (n = 38)
Age, (months) mean (SD)	58.3 (14.6)	59.1 (13.4)	58.7 (13.8)
Gender, N (%)			
Female	3 (15.8)	3 (15.8)	6 (15.8)
Male	16 (84.2)	16 (84.2)	32 (84.2)
Educational Placement, N (%)			
Regular classroom	3 (15.8)	4 (21.1)	7 (18.4)
Special education classroom	10 (52.6)	7 (36.8)	17 (44.7)
Preschool	3 (15.8)	6 (31.6)	9 (23.7)
None	3 (15.8)	2 (10.5)	5 (13.2)
Number of adults in the home, N (%)			
1	2 (10.5)	0 (0)	2 (5.3)
2	15 (79.0)	16 (84.2)	31 (81.6)
3	2 (10.5)	3 (15.8)	5 (13.1)

A portion of the evaluation's results can be shown in Example 9.4.

Example 9.4 A Table of Statistical Results Comparing Program EAT and Parent Education at Baseline, 12 Weeks, and 16 Weeks

	Program EAT[a] (N = 19)	Parent Education (N = 19)	Adjusted Mean Difference (95% CI)[b]	P-Value[c] (Effect Size)[d]
Food Selectivity Score[e]				
Baseline	14.52 (3.70)[e]	15.22 (1.85)		
Week 12	14.21 (1.48)	14.38 (1.98)	−6.15 (−10.74, −1.56)	0.010 (0.60)
Week 16	13.51 (2.11)	15.05 (1.18)	−7.04 (−12.57, −1.51)	0.014 (0.68)
Disruptive Mealtime Behavior Score				
Baseline	10.95 (94.64)	11.63 (5.02)		
Week 12	8.05 (2.04)	11.72 (3.97)	−3.43 (−5.38, −1.47)	<0.001 (0.72)
Week 16	8.87 (3.89)	12.57 (4.24)	−3.43 (−6.16, −0.69)	0.016 (0.72)

[a] Data is presented as least-square means (SD) from mixed model.
[b] Adjusted mean differences = difference of least square means from mixed models conditioned on baseline score.
[c] P-value from mixed model condition on baseline score – value of p<0.05 are statistically significant.
[d] Effect size calculated from the absolute value of the adjusted means differences divided by the pooled standard deviation at baseline.
[e] Scores on the Child Nutrition Test, 20 = Negative behavior; 1 = positive

Evaluation tables follow certain guidelines:

- Tables display columns and rows of numbers, percentages, scores, and statistical test results. They can become very busy, so it is important to make sure that they remain readable. Decide how many columns and rows you can include and keep the table readable.

Each table should have a title that summarizes its research design, purpose, and content. For example: "A Pragmatic randomized controlled trial to evaluate the effectiveness and cost effectiveness of a multi-component intervention to reduce substance use and risk-taking behaviour in adolescents involved in the criminal justice system" or The Effect of Music Therapy on Parent–Infant Bonding Among Infants Born Preterm: A Randomized Clinical Trial."

- When you use a term that may be confusing, define it. Set off definitions with asterisks or superscripts.
- Columns are independent variables, such as group.
- Many evaluators use only horizontal lines in tables. Use vertical lines sparingly, especially if you also use horizontal lines.
- Include the sample size and differentiate among numbers, percentages, and other statistics.

The Abstract

The abstract of an evaluation report is usually quite brief: between 200 and 300 words. Its purpose is to present the evaluation's main objectives, methods, and findings. The following topics are usually addressed in the abstract, although the amount of detail about each topic varies:

Objective: In one or two sentences, tell the purpose of the evaluation.

Design: Using standard terminology, name the design (e.g., *randomized controlled trial* or *true experiment*; *nonrandomized trial* or *quasi-experiment*; *survey*). Describe any unique feature of the design, such as the use of blinding.

Participants: Describe the characteristics of the participants, including the numbers of participants in the experimental and control groups, demographics (such as age, income, and health status), region of the country, and size of facility (such as hospital, clinic, school). Describe any unique features of the participants, such as their location or special health characteristics.

Main outcome measures: Describe the main outcomes and how they were measured. Describe any unique features of the measures, use their proper names if appropriate, and include any special notes on reliability or validity.

Results or findings: For each major dependent variable, give the results.

Conclusions: In one or two sentences, explain what the results mean. Did the program work? Is it applicable to other participants?

Example 9.5 provides an illustration of an annotated abstract.

Example 9.5 An Annotated Abstract for an Evaluation of an Online Education Program for Older Adults

Objective: To develop and evaluate an online program to improve older adults' skills in identifying high-quality web-based health information.

Design: Mixed methods: surveys and randomized, control trial. We conducted focus groups and individual interviews to collect data on older adults' preferences for online instruction and information. We used the findings to develop, pilot test, and evaluate an interactive website which was grounded in health behavior change models, adult education, and website construction.

Programs: A newly designed web-based program, *Your Health Online* (the experimental group) compared to an existing online slide show, *Evaluating Health Information*.

Setting: Community senior center.

Participants: 300 people 55 years of age and older who used the internet for health information at least once in the last 12 months; 30 people participated in program development; 185 were assigned to the new or existing program.

Main outcome measures: Newly designed measures of usability, satisfaction, and knowledge; The Senior Self-Efficacy Report.

Results: Experimental participants assigned significantly higher ratings of usability and learning (p = .003) to the new site than controls did to their tutorial although no differences were found in self-efficacy or knowledge. Experimental participants reported that participation was likely to improve future searches (p = .02).

Conclusion: A website such as *Your Health Online* is feasible for use among many older adults, and it contains useful and usable information. People who work with older adults should consider how to obtain and integrate web-based instruction into their practices.

Word count (including subheadings is 240).

The Executive Summary

The evaluation report's executive summary provides all potential users with an easy-to-read digest of the evaluation's major purposes, methods, findings, and recommendations. Executive summaries are relatively brief, usually from three to 15 pages in length. Evaluation funders nearly always require that reports include such summaries, and they frequently specify the number of pages expected.

Three rules should govern your preparation of an executive summary for your evaluation report:

1. Include the important purposes, methods, findings, and recommendations.
2. Avoid the use of jargon. If necessary, define terms. For example:
   Poor:
   We investigated *concurrent validity by correlating scores* on Measure A with those on Measure B.
   Better:
   Concurrent validity means that two measures produce the same results. We examined the statistical relationship between scores on Measures A and B to investigate their concurrent validity.
3. Use active verbs.
   Poor:
   The use of health care services *was found* by the evaluation to be more frequent in people 45 years of age or younger.
   Better:
   The evaluation found more frequent use of services by people 45 years of age or younger.
   Poor:
   It is recommended that the prevention of prematurity be the focus of prenatal care education.
   Better:
   The ABC Group recommends that the prevention of prematurity be the focus of prenatal care education.

As you prepare the executive summary, you should provide information on the program, evaluation, findings, conclusions, and recommendations:

The program or intervention: Describe the program's purposes and objectives, settings, and unique features. Consider answering questions like these:

- During which years did the program take place?
- Who were the funders?
- How did the program differ from others that have similar purposes?
- How great was the need for the program?

The evaluation: Present an overview of the purposes of the evaluation, describe the evaluation framework, describe and justify the evaluation questions/hypotheses and choice of evidence of effectiveness, quality, and value; explain the design and sample; discuss the outcomes and how they were measured; and explain the main analytic methods. Consider answering questions like these:

- What were the purposes of the evaluation?
- On what basis were the evaluation questions selected?
- How were the evidence of effectiveness, quality, and value chosen and justified and by whom?
- Were the evaluation methods unique in any way?
- Who performed the evaluation?
- During which years did the evaluation take place?
- For whom are the evaluation's findings and recommendations most applicable?

The findings: Give the answers to the evaluation questions.
Consider answering questions like these:

- Is the program likely to be sustainable over time?
- Who benefited most (and least) from participation?

Conclusions: Tell whether the program solved the problem it was designed to solve. Was the program effective? Are the findings consistent with those of evaluations of similar programs? For whom is the program most likely to be effective?

Recommendations: Tell other evaluators, researchers, and policy makers about the implications of the evaluation. Explain the changes to the program that can make it more effective. Describe the participants who are most likely to need the program in the future. Describe ways to improve future programs and evaluations.

REVIEWING THE REPORT FOR QUALITY: CONSORT AND TREND

Program evaluations that are submitted to academic journals are increasingly required to complete a reporting checklist whose objective is to ensure the report's comprehensiveness and transparency. Perhaps the most famous is the Consolidated Standards of Reporting Trials (*CONSORT*). The CONSORT Statement consists of standards for *reporting* on randomized controlled trials. The Statement is available in several languages and has been endorsed by prominent medical, clinical, and psychological journals. The CONSORT Statement, widely adopted in 2010, is continuously being updated, so before using it, the evaluator must check for recent editions.

Figure 9.2 contains brief excerpts from the CONSORT Statement.

Section/Topic	Item No	Checklist item	Reported on Page No.
Title and abstract			
	1a	Identification as a randomized trial in the title	
	1b	Structured summary of trial design, methods, results, and conclusions (for specific guidance see CONSORT for abstracts)	
Introduction			
Background and objectives	2a	Scientific background and explanation of rationale	
	2b	Specific objectives or hypotheses	
Methods			
Trial design	3a	Description of trial design (such as parallel, factorial) including allocation ratio	
	3b	Important changes to methods after trial commencement (such as eligibility criteria), with reasons	
Participants	4a	Eligibility criteria for participants	
	4b	Settings and locations where the data were collected	
Interventions	5	The interventions for each group with sufficient details to allow replication, including how and when they were actually administered	
Outcomes	6a	Completely defined pre-specified primary and secondary outcome measures, including how and when they were assessed	
	6b	Any changes to trial outcomes after the trial commenced, with reasons	
Sample size	7a	How sample size was determined	
	7b	When applicable, explanation of any interim analyses and stopping guidelines	
Randomization:			
Sequence generation	8a	Method used to generate the random allocation sequence	
	8b	Type of randomization; details of any restriction (such as blocking and block size)	
Allocation concealment	9	Mechanism used to implement the random allocation sequence (such as sequentially numbered containers), describing any steps taken to conceal the sequence until interventions were assigned	

Figure 9.2 Brief Excerpts from the CONSORT 2010 Checklist of Information to Include When Reporting a Randomized Trial

Table 9.1 Brief Portion of the Transparent Reporting of Evaluations with Non-Randomized Designs (TREND) Statement: Descriptions of Information on Baseline Data and Equivalence of Groups that Should Be Reported

Baseline Data	14	Baseline demographic and clinical characteristics of participants in each study condition
		Baseline characteristics for each study condition relevant to specific disease prevention research
		Baseline comparisons of those lost to follow-up and those retained, overall and by study condition
		Comparison between study population at baseline and target population of interest
Baseline equivalence	15	Data on study group equivalence at baseline and statistical methods used to control for baseline differences

Not all evaluations are RCT's, and the *TREND* (Transparent Reporting of Evaluations with Nonrandomized Designs) Statement (Centers for Disease Control, www.cdc.gov/trendstatement/index.html) was designed for these studies. Table 9.1 contains the portion of the TREND Statement that is concerned with the factors that evaluators must include when reporting on baseline differences.

Although CONSORT and TREND were developed by health researchers, other fields such as psychology and substance abuse have begun to require that evaluators demonstrate that their reports have accounted for each item on the appropriate checklist. Reporting guidelines for many study types, including qualitative research can be found at www.equator-network.org/reporting-guidelines.

ORAL PRESENTATIONS

An oral presentation consists of an account of some or all of the evaluation's objectives, methods, and findings. Most commonly, oral evaluation reports take the form of "slide" presentations. If you need to prepare an oral presentation, regardless of its duration, the following recommendations can be helpful.

Recommendations for Slide Presentations

1. *Do the talking and explaining and let the audience listen.* Use slides to focus the audience's attention on the key points of your talk. Do not require audience members to read and listen at the same time.

Poor:

Reliability

A reliable measure is one that is relatively free from measurement error. Because of this error, individuals' obtained scores are different from their true scores. In some cases, the error results from the measure itself: It may be difficult to understand or poorly administered.

Better:

Reliable Measures

Reliable measures are relatively free of error.
  Two causes of error are common:

- The measure is hard to understand.
- The measure is poorly administered.

The second of the two slides above is better than the first because the listener can more easily keep the main points in view without being distracted by a lot of reading requirements. If your objective is to have the audience read something, a handout (and the time to read it) is more appropriate than a slide.

2. *Make sure that each slide has a title.*
3. *During the talk, address the talk's purposes and the evaluation's purposes, main methods, main results, conclusions, and recommendations.*
4. *Keep tables and figures simple.* Explain the meaning of each table and figure, the title, the column and row headings, and the statistics. Consider this table headed "Knowledge: How the CAPs and the Control Compare."
   Consider saying something like this:

> The next slide compares the knowledge of children in CAP with those in the controls. We used the CAP Test, in which higher scores are better, and the highest score is 50 points.
>   As you can see [if possible, point to the appropriate place on the screen], children who are 4 and 5 did significantly better in CAP. We found no differences in children who were 6 and 7.

5. *Check all slides carefully for typographic errors.*
6. *Avoid the use of abbreviations and acronyms unless you are certain that your audience members will know what they mean.* In these examples, the acronym CAP

Knowledge: How the CAPs and the Control Programs Compare

Age	Experimental	Control
	Scores	Scores
4	45	22*
5	46	20**
6	33	29
7	35	32

HIGHER SCORES ARE BETTER
STATISTICAL SIGNIFICANCE: $*p = .03$; $**p = .001$

(Notice that no decimals are used in the table above; numbers should be rounded to the nearest whole number.)

was explained in the first slide. If necessary, you should explain and define each abbreviation and acronym.

7. *Outline or write out what you plan to say.*
8. *Rehearse the presentation before you create the final copies of the slides.* Then rehearse again. The purpose of the first rehearsal is to make sure that the talk is logical, that the spelling on all slides is correct, and that the arrangement of words, figures, and tables is meaningful. The second rehearsal is to make sure that you haven't introduced new errors.
9. *Ensure that the slides are easy to see.* Horizontal placement is better than vertical. All potential audience members should be able to see the slides. In advance of the talk, check the room, the seating plan, and the place where you will stand.
10. *Use humor and rhetorical questions to engage listeners.* Typical rhetorical questions are given in three of the slides above: Who was in CAP? How was the information collected? Do the results fit?
11. *Allow the audience one to two minutes to view each slide.*
12. *Be consistent in using complete sentences or sentence fragments or parts of speech within a given slide.*

Poor:

Implementation Evaluation

- Teachers were given a one-week in-service course
- Random observation of their classes
- There were two observers.
- 10% of all classes
- Kappa = .80, which is high

Better:

Implementation Evaluation

Teachers participated in a one-week in-service course.
Two observers monitored 10% of classes at random for program implementation.
The agreement between observers was high: Kappa = .80.

The first of these two slides mixes sentence fragments ("random observation of their classes") and full sentences, whereas the second uses only full sentences.

13. *If you have downtime with no appropriate slides, use fillers.* These are often opaque, blank slides or slides showing only the title of the presentation. Consider using cartoons as fillers but be careful in their use: They can be distracting in the middle of a talk.
14. *Use handouts to summarize information and provide technical details and references.* Make sure that your name, the name of the presentation, and the date are on each page of every handout. Do not distribute handouts until you are finished speaking unless you plan to refer to them during your presentation. If possible, post your slides online to make them accessible to listeners.
15. *When you create your slides, use upper- and lowercase letters in the text; in general, this is easier to read than text that is all uppercase.*
16. *Make sure that you discuss in your talk all the information that is displayed on the screen.*

17. *Be careful not to overwhelm your audience with animation, graphics, and sound.* Also, do not assume that you can routinely use graphics or other materials downloaded from the Internet. A great deal of the information accessible there is protected by copyright.
18. *Use no more than four colors per slide.* If you are unsure about which colors to use, consider using the slide presentation colors that are preselected by the software you use to create the slides. Yellow or white letters on royal blue are easy to see and read.

POSTERS

A poster is a visual printed summary of the evaluation that is designed to be read and understood without oral explanation. Using a relatively large print out, you rely on short text sections and give the results as bullet points. Most evaluation posters also incorporate graphical elements to help illustrate key points. Remember: A poster is not a thesis or journal article, so don't try to cram all the details onto it. A casual viewer should be able to get the message in three to five minutes and read all the text in no more than ten minutes.

The poster is a report, so be sure to include the introduction and study objectives, methods (including research design, programs, sampling, and data analysis), results, and conclusions. You may also want to include an abstract, acknowledgments, and references.

A poster should have a main title that's readable from 25 feet away. People will be wandering through the poster session, so you need to catch their eye from a distance. A general rule is to use a 72-point type and a common font such as Times New Roman or Arial for your poster title and to use a smaller size of the same font for the section titles. Use a simple color scheme. Don't distract people by using too many different colors, fonts, and font sizes. A general rule is 60% images and 40% text. Make sure the images are 150 dpi or larger.

Think about how you plan to print your poster before you design it. Because not every printing option offers the same paper dimensions and because larger poster sizes generally cost more to print, first choose the paper size for printing, and then design your poster accordingly. Then check with your printing vendor to find out whether you should be aware of any specific limitations or guidelines.

Microsoft PowerPoint is a relatively easy-to-use tool for creating posters although many other programs are available that have multiple design features and produce excellent results.

With a little searching, you can find free online templates for setting up your poster. For instance, several online sites have collections of free PowerPoint (.ppt and. pptx native formats) research poster templates. You download the appropriate PowerPoint poster template, add text, images, and graphics, and send it back to the company for printing. The University of North Carolina's website has many excellent tips on poster presentations (https://gradschool.unc.edu/academics/resources/postertips.html) as do Washington State University (https://posters.wsu.edu/making-posters-with-powerpoint) and New York University (https://guides.nyu.edu/posters).

A typical academic poster that reports on the impact of patient education on COVID-19 care is shown in Figure 9.3.

Impact of Patient Education on Preferences for Extracorporeal Membrane Oxygenation in COVID Care

Ethan D. Borre, PhD;[1] Matthew L. Maciejewski, PhD;[1,2] Arlene Fink, PhD;[3] Melissa Burnside, MD;[1] J. Todd Purves, MD, PhD;[1] Charles D Scales Jr., MD, MSHS;[1] Eddy Fan, MD, PhD,[4] Bhawandip Sandhu, HBSc, CCP, CPC, MHM;[4] Kevin Pignone;[5] Caroline Palmer;[1] Carrington Webb;[6] Dana S. Guggenheim;[1] Yuqi Zhang, MD[1]
[1]Duke University School of Medicine, [2]Durham VA HSR&D, [3]University of California Los Angeles, [4]University of Toronto, [5]University of North Carolina-Chapel Hill

Department of Population Health Sciences
Duke University School of Medicine

BACKGROUND

- Extracorporeal membrane oxygenation (ECMO) is a scarce and critical resource for COVID care.
- Potential knowledge gap between patients and providers about benefits and risks of ECMO for COVID care.
- Hypothesis: an educational intervention would align ECMO preferences between patients and providers; providers will be more selective about recommending ECMO than patients.

OBJECTIVE

To assess 1) concordance in ECMO care preferences between patients and providers and 2) the effect of an ECMO educational intervention on patient knowledge and preferences.

METHODS

- Recruited outpatient primary care patients at Duke Primary care, randomized into two groups: 1) Video+Survey, and 2) Survey Only.
- Video+Survey participants watched brief video on the purpose, benefits, and risks of ECMO.
- Both groups completed an identical survey on ECMO knowledge and care preferences.
- Providers were administered the survey alone.
- Preference questions varied by age, functional ability, and comorbidity. For example:
  - *Jane is 35 years old and lives at home by herself independently. She recently became sick with COVID19 and is currently in the hospital with a breathing tube. She displays no improvement after 5 days on a breathing machine.*
- Logistic regression to predict the probability of ECMO agreement for each of 7 patient scenarios between the two patient groups. Second logistic regression comparing all patients and providers.

RESULTS

Figure 1. Study Flow Diagram.

Figure 2. Screenshots from the Educational Video.

Table 1. Percent Agreement that ECMO be Provided Among Patients and Providers.

	All Patients (n=41)	Providers (n=20)	p-value
Answering all 4 ECMO knowledge questions correctly	43%	58%	0.28
35-year-old female, lives independently	84%	88%	0.62
35-year-old female, lives independently, takes 3 pills/day for diabetes + high BP	93%	92%	0.91
35-year-old female, because of weakness in arms and legs, she needs an aide to help her bathe and dress	85%	84%	0.95
35-year-old female, because of weakness in arms and legs, she needs an aide to help her bathe and dress, takes 3 pills/day for diabetes and high BP	87%	71%	0.14
65-year-old female, lives independently	94%	90%	0.53
65-year-old female, lives independently, takes 3 pills/day for diabetes and high BP	89%	84%	0.56
65-year-old female, because of weakness in arms and legs, she needs an aide to help her bathe and dress, takes 3 pills/day for diabetes and high BP	84%	41%	0.003

Figure 3. Unadjusted Proportion of Participants Endorsing ECMO in Each Patient Scenario

- Among patients, there was high endorsement that ECMO be provided for all patients.
- Adjusted results showed no significant difference in ECMO preferences between patients who did or did not view educational video.

REGRESSION RESULTS

- Patients Randomized to Survey Only were significantly less likely to answer all four ECMO knowledge questions correctly (17%) compared to the Video+Survey (64%, p=0.02).
- For the highest risk patients, patients endorsed ECMO consideration significantly more frequently (predicted probability: 84%) than providers (41%, p=0.003).
- All regressions controlled for: age, gender, race, education, and marital status.

LIMITATIONS

- Patients were limited to primary care and age 50+.
- Significant differences in history of family member of friend hospitalized for COVID between the two patient groups.

CONCLUSIONS

- An educational video can increase patient knowledge of the benefits and risks of ECMO.
- There are differences in ECMO care preferences between patients and providers for high-risk patients.
- These differences may be addressable by targeted patient education.

DISCLOSURES
This research was funded by the National Institutes of Health. (F30 DC019846), the Duke National Clinician Scholar Program and VA HSR&D (RCS 10-391).

Figure 9.3 A Poster Reporting on the Impact of Patient Education on COVID-19 Care

EXERCISES: CHAPTER 9

Exercise 1

Directions

Review the following slide prepared as a visual aid for an oral evaluation presentation and, if necessary, improve it.

A **stratified random sample** is one in which the population is divided into subgroups or "strata," and a random sample is then selected from each group. For example, in a program to teach women about options for treatment for breast cancer, the evaluator can sample from several subgroups including women of differing ages (under 19 years, 20 to 30, 31 to 35, over 35) and income (high, medium, low).

Exercise 2

Directions

The following table compares boys' and girls' sleeping patterns. Following the table is an explanation of the data in the table. The explanation contains two errors. What are they?

Variable	N	Mean (s.d.)	P-value[a]	Hours of sleep per night (%)			P-value[b]
				8	8–10.9	11	
Gender			0.004				0.02
Boys	2193	9.6 (1.4)		6.7	48.2	45.1	
Girls	2258	9.7 (1.4)		7.2	44.0	48.8	
Socio-economic level			<0.001				<0.001
A (wealthiest)	164	9.3 (1.3)		15.9	47.0	37.2	
B	697	9.5 (1.3)		9.1	49.9	41.1	
C	1513	9.7 (1.4)		6.9	46.7	46.5	
D	1719	9.8 (1.4)		5.2	44.9	49.9	
E	308	9.9 (1.6)		6.8	42.2	51.0	
Maternal education (year)			<0.001				<0.001
9	1086	9.6 (1.4)		9.7	46.2	44.2	
5–8	2124	9.7 (1.4)		6.3	47.3	46.4	
1–4	1133	9.8 (1.4)		5.7	44.3	50.0	
0	101	10.0 (1.4)		3.8	39.0	57.1	

Variable	N	Mean (s.d.)	P-value[a]	Hours of sleep per night (%)			P-value[b]
				8	8–10.9	11	
Birth order			0.09				0.1
1	1558	9.6 (1.4)		8.1	46.7	45.2	
2	1241	9.7 (1.4)		5.7	46.4	47.9	
3	799	9.7 (1.4)		7.0	47.2	45.7	
4	358	9.8 (1.4)		7.0	40.7	52.3	
5	495	9.8 (1.4)		6.1	45.3	48.6	
Birthweight (g)			0.015				0.017
2500	4053	9.7 (1.4)		7.2	46.2	46.6	
<2500	398	9.9 (1.3)		3.8	44.8	51.4	
Maternal BMI (kg/m2)			0.6				0.8
Normal weight	3339	9.7 (1.4)		6.8	46.7	46.6	

Abbreviation: BMI, body mass index.

[a] One-way analysis of variance.
[b] χ^2-Test.

Explanation of Table:

The table presents unadjusted data on sleep duration. Boys slept, on average, significantly more than girls ($P<0.05$). Socio-economic level was inversely associated with sleep duration, and so was birthweight ($P<0.02$). No significant associations were detected for maternal pre-pregnancy BMI or parity, nor for gestational age, maternal smoking and alcohol intake during pregnancy (data not shown). χ^2-Tests confirmed a significantly increased proportion of adolescents with longer sleep duration in girls, in adolescents from poorer backgrounds or of lower level of maternal education, and with lower birthweight. Obesity was associated with maternal social status, with prevalence values from richest to poorest social status groups being 17.1, 16.7, 13.6, 9.0 and 2.9% respectively.

SUGGESTED READINGS

Butcher, N.J., Monsour, A., Mew, E.J., et al. (2022). Guidelines for Reporting Outcomes in Trial Reports: The CONSORT-Outcomes 2022 Extension. JAMA, *328*(22): 2252–2264.

Suggested Websites

University of North Carolina Graduate School: Academic Presentations and Posters
https://gradschool.unc.edu/academics/resources/postertips.html

Karina Adcock: How to Make an Academic Poster in PowerPoint
www.youtube.com/watch?v=_WnhoIbfcoM

Washington State University: Making Posters with PowerPoint
https://posters.wsu.edu/making-posters-with-powerpoint

ANSWERS TO EXERCISES: CHAPTER 9

Exercise 1

The slide asks the audience to do too much reading. Also, the slide title should be more informative. Two slides will be better:

---

1. Stratified Random Sampling

- Population is divided into subgroups or strata.
- Random samples are selected from each stratum.

Stratified Random Sampling Example

	INCOME		
AGE IN YEARS	**High**	**Medium**	**Low**
Under 19			
20-30			
31-35			
35 and older			

Exercise 2

The errors are:

1. Boys slept on average, significantly *less* than girls ($P<.05$).
2. *No* significant associations were detected for maternal prepregnancy, BMI, or parity, nor for gestational age, maternal smoking, and alcohol intake during pregnancy.

Note to index: page numbers in *italics* refer to information in figures; page numbers in **bold** refer to information in tables.

effectiveness, quality and value
50–9; and expert consultation 54–5;
literature reviews 52, 57–8; sources of
52–8; and statistical significance 43,
52–4; structure, process and outcome
51–2; unbiased 43
evidence statements 50
exclusion criteria (samples) 98
executive summaries 190–1
expectancy, as threat to internal validity 87
experimental evaluation design 66, 68–70 *see
also* randomized controlled trials (RCT)
experimental groups 69, 71–4
experimental studies 14
experiments, true 18
expert advice 52
expert consultation 54–6
expert panels 55–6
explanatory variables *see* independent variables
exploratory questions 47
external validity 86–8

face validity 132
factorial designs 81–2, *82*, 85
factors (in factorial designs) 81–2
field notes 174, 176
figures, in evaluation reports 186, *187*
findings 6, 29
flow charts 186, *187*
FMS scores 4
focus groups 174
formative evaluation data 12–13
frameworks *see* evaluation frameworks
funding agencies 12, 13

goals, of programs 45–6
group assignments 78
groups: creating (matching) 69; experimental
69, 71–4

Hawthorne effect 87
healthy eating programs 4
historical studies *see* retrospective (historical)
studies
history, as threat to internal validity 86
homogeneity (Cronbach's coefficient alpha) 131
human subjects, and ethics 1
hypotheses: identifying 7–8; null hypothesis
53, 104–5, **105**, 168; and program
evaluation questions 43, 45, 47
hypothesis testing 105, **105**, 167, 168–9

implementation evaluations *see* process
(implementation) evaluations
inclusion criteria (samples) 98
incomparable participants 78

independent variables 59, 77, 163, **166**–**7**; and
confounding variables 78; factors 81;
and inclusion/exclusion criteria 98; in
stratified sampling 102
index 134
informed consent/forms 23–6, 29
institutional review boards (IRB) 21–4 *see
also* ethics boards
instrumentation, as threat to internal
validity 86
instruments (measures) 134, 137
intention-to-treat analysis (ITT) 154
interdisciplinary teams (of evaluators) 5, 30
interim data 13
internal consistency 131
internal validity 86–8
internet 26–8
interrater reliability 131
interruption, as threat to internal validity 87
intervention alignment 19
interviews 117; computer-assisted 117–18;
field notes 174, 176; qualitative data
16; transcripts 173, 176
intrarater reliability 131
IRB approval *see* institutional review boards
(IRB)

kappa statistic 149–51

last observation carried forward (LOCF) 154
likelihood ratios *see* risk ratios
literature reviews: "best available" literature
123; as data source 118–24; as
evidence 52, 57–8; extracting
information 123–4; non-peer-reviewed
literature 125; published reports 118,
125; search terms 119, *120*, *121*, *122*
logical connections (measurement charts) 138
logistic regression analysis 153–4
longitudinal studies *see* prospective
(longitudinal) studies

matching: creating groups 69; in
nonrandomized controlled trials 77–8
maturation, as threat to internal validity 86
mean (average) calculation 54
measurement charts 138–40, **139**
measurement error 130
measures 130, 134–8
median 164
mediator variables *see* confounding variables
meta-analysis 119, 177–8
metrics 130, 134
misconduct *see* research misconduct
missing data / nonresponse: rules for 176; and
statistical methods 152–4

For Product Safety Concerns and Information please contact our EU
representative GPSR@taylorandfrancis.com Taylor & Francis Verlag GmbH,
Kaufingerstraße 24, 80331 München, Germany

Printed and bound by CPI Group (UK) Ltd, Croydon, CR0 4YY
08/06/2025
01897009-0014